CYCLES IN MEDICAL ASTROLOGY

WILLIAM MORRIS, PHD

Cycles in Medical Astrology

William Morris, PhD

© 2018 33Publishing

Back cover photography Christina McHugh
https://www.mchughphotography.com/

First Edition; First Printing

2018 33 17 16 15 14 13 6 5 4 3 2 1

ISBN-13: 978-0-9831026-2-5

In the heart of the sky, planetary movements arise and depart while humans wander this world in relationship to one another, the earth, and the heavens. Each life arises from the ancestral gene pool and culminates, returning to source.

~ William Morris

GRATITUDE

To the east, I bow in deep gratitude to the masters who have influenced the features of this book. It is the subtle currents of inspiration from the Shang, Zhou, and Han dynasties that brought me to the realizations of cycles in relation to medicine. In particular, I honor those beings in spirit who are with me through their writings: Bian Que, Lao Zi, Huang Di, Zhong Zhong Jing, and Shen Nung, more recently, John HF Shen and Leon Hammer.

To the west, I bow in deep gratitude to the masters who have influenced the medicinal features of this book through the inner temple: Pythagoras, Asclepius, Galen, and Hippocrates.

To the south and north, I make the deepest bow in gratitude to ancient and contemporary masters who have influenced the astrological features of this work. Graciousness extends to my teachers, in astrology especially Lee Lehman, Marc Boney, KN Rao, Mark Jones, Scott Silverman, and David Cochrane who encourage and support my efforts. Also – gratitude towards Alfred Witte, Reinhold Ebertin, Guido Bonatti, William Lilly, and Nicholas Culpeper, who guide in spirit and in word the development of my practice.

In the center are my family and friends. My beloved wife, Theresa Lee, and my children, Joshua, Solena, and Zoe. And my dear friend Scott Silverman who is always supportive of my astrological works.

CONTENTS

OPENING

My greatest passion is weaving mystical, musical and medical disciplines. As I wiped the sweat from my brow after a night's work playing jazz, a fan explained to me the ecliptic and the movement of planets through the sky. Then, since exploring the depths of Dane Rudhyar's, *The Astrology of Personality*, I have not looked back. I studied with every astrologer possible from Marion March to Eileen Nauman, KN Rao, Rob Hand, Rob Zoller, Olivia Barclay, David Cochrane, and Lee Lehman.

Seeking the path that connects, I recognized that Western music has twelve keys and astrology has twelve signs. Further, the channel systems of acupuncture are twelve. These connections have fascinated me for the past 38 years as I have worked with them in my practice where I have guided the use of herbs, acupuncture, and healing music through astrology.

There is no question, that for me, astrologically informed clinical practice has greater power than my practice without it. One example is the richness and depth of dialog between my client and myself produces better results as the vision of the client's shared experience opens a new field of possibilities. On a practical level, I look at the synodic motion of the planets relative to the Nodal Axis of the Moon as a tool for facilitating an integral level of personal growth, healing, and spiritual evolution.

In 1987, I discovered Robert Carl Jansky's book, *Astrology, Nutrition & Health* [1]. In it he described a medical technique using the north and south nodes of the Moon as a tool for correlating anatomy with the astrological chart. This awakened knowledge for me and has provided seed for this book.

INTRODUCTION

In this book, I present tools for analyzing the chart in relationship to cyclic motions. Treatment strategies are also provided. The cycles of movement focus on the day, month, and year, but most importantly the Moon's Nodes as whole systems for exploring and treating the human condition.

Treatment strategies are presented that direct, guide, supplement, or remove obstructions from the cyclic movement for the achievement of one's goals, but more importantly, for one's own good.

LOCATION, PROCESS AND SEVERITY

Location and process are at the heart of medicine. 'My knee is broken,' tells us what and where. If there is arthritis of the knee, a pattern of signs and symptoms are explored. Inflammation has a pattern of heat, pain, redness, and swelling. Thus, the Moon conjunct Mars in Capricorn describes heat, pain, redness, and swelling in the knees. Similarly, asthma is located in the lungs it may be severe, and may or may not be associated with phlegm.

SIGNS AND SYMPTOMS

Signs are those phenomena which the practitioner observes. These include physical examination, labs, and imaging. The symptom is the client's experience of their condition.

For the medical astrologer, signs include what which is in the heavens. The symptom often signals the location of a problem; both medical and oracular arts depend upon signs which form recognizable patterns.

As the famous Indian astrologer K.N. Rao says, and I paraphrase, "We are seeking confluence at the location where the rivers meet."

The confluence is that moment when the signs and symptoms are all aligned in the same direction, and a sense of reliability increases. Heres an example of confluence which may also be described as coherence, the person:

- easily gest cold
- has a predominance of cold signs (earth and water)
- was born in winter at midnight on a new Moon (cycles!).

These signs and symptoms coherently point towards cold. This is a more reliable confluence of signs than when they are disparate conditions where the client is very hot and red, but the astrological signs are cold and dry, as with Saturn and earth signs.

APPLICABILITY OF THE METHODS IN THIS BOOK

The methods in this book may be used for any chart technique. I use the natal chart for constitutional concerns and tendencies towards disease. I also erect a chart for the moment of the consultation. A chart may be calculated for the onset of a condition, and is called the *decumbiture*.[1] The most commonly used charts in my practice are the nativity and the consultation chart.

Not addressed in this book are other charting methods to which the tools in this book may also be applied. Electional charts[2] are used for diagnostics, procedures, and starting therapeutic regimens such as diets or exercise. Synastry can be used to explore the relationship between the practitioner and the client.

Astrology is one of the best tools for prognostication according to K.S. Charak, MD. Such charts are the planetary period (Time

---

[1]   Decumbiture refers to a chart calculated for the time that a client lays down with a disease. In todays climate of chronic degenerative disease, a precise time of disease onset can be difficult.

[2]   Also called inception charts.

Lord), transit, solar return, solar arc, progressed charts, and critical day charts. Please see Appendix V for definitions of the terms.

AN EXTREMELY BRIEF HISTORY OF MEDICAL ASTROLOGY

The *Upanishads* discuss a form of the Zodiac Person as the grand cosmos forms Shiva's body. This heavenly body, called the *Kalapurusha,* describes the embodiment of time as the relationship between the signs and anatomy. The *Upanishads* are sacred Hindu texts that provide a substantive cosmology for the assignment of heavenly observations to human anatomy.

Western tradition describes cosmic anatomy as *Melothesia, Homo Signorum* or the Zodiac Man, which I call the Zodiac Person, not for political correctness, but for accuracy.

The idea of *Melothesia* likely arose during the Hellenistic period, as the preceding Babylonian period used decans (*dodecatemoria*) for the assignment of anatomy to the portions of the zodiac [2]. The use of the term *Homo Signorum* first appeared later in an almanac by one Petrus de Cacia circa 1300 CE according to Cox [3]. It then became commonly used in almanacs, which were a tool for disseminating knowledge related to medical astrology [4].

These concepts of - *Melothesia, Homo Signorum* and *Kalapurusha* - are terms for assigning anatomy to astrological signs and houses. In this book, I address the head and tail of the dragon - the Moon's Nodes - as a basis for anatomical references.

Ever an array of cultural perspectives on astrological anatomy, there are common threads. This is particularly true when comparing Hellenistic astrology with that of India. Both use planetary periods, known to the Greeks as time lord systems, and to the

Indians as *dasas*.[3] Classical Greek culture finds root not only within pre-Indo-European cultures of the Mother Goddess of Neolithic Europe, but also Mesopotamia, the Middle East, Egypt, and India [5]. Similarly, India absorbed western thought during the same time frame. Nowhere is connection more obvious than the assignment of the liver to the planet Jupiter.

Humoral thought is the most glaring example of cross-cultural pollination [6]. It is present in Greece, Europe, India, China, Tibet, and First Nation practices of the Americas.

Greeks may have influenced the Chinese conceptions of the humors surrounding concepts of hot, cold, moist, and dry [7]. While the Greeks name four elements, they also identify *pneuma*, which is synonymous with the Chinese term *qi* and the Ayurvedic term *prana*. All are commensurate with breath and *vitality* – a core feature of the Sun in medical astrology.[4]

Thus, astrological practices extend into the shrouded mists of time, deep into the origins of humanity. The tools of astrology became codified during the Stoic and Hellenistic periods. But, they are not so far distant from the types of thinking used in contemporary Chinese medical practices, with their humoral bases. The methods I am about to present combine astrological practices from earlier periods with trends and breakthroughs in contemporary thought. Before I describe these methods in more detail, I would like to explore the contributions of the Greeks to humoral thought.

---

[3] A single planetary period creates a backdrop for transits to be understood in better detail than through inquiry into transits alone. I learned to combine multiple planetary period systems from KN Rao. When they are congruent with each other, the odds of accuracy are increased.

[4] Vitalism is essential to the effective practice of medical astrology. It was the cultures that built their medical philosophy on vitalism that consistently applied astromedical thought.

GREEK THOUGHT IN THE HUMORS

Empedocles, of the Greek Island Kos, might be rightfully considered to be the source of the medical cults of Asclepius. He viewed the universe as composed of and driven by various distributions of heat, cold, moisture and dryness [8].

The title 'Asclepiad' suggests that Hippocrates took Oath in the fraternity of Apollo. God of medicine and possessor of the serpent-entwined staff, Asclepius parented both Hygeia and Panacea, as well as, all the healing disciplines. When the daughters of Asclepius attended the temples, Hygeia brought cleanliness and purification while Panacea brought medicinals. This book focuses on medicinals and interventions more so than hygiene.

The symbol of the single serpent was associated with the temple dream healers and removers of parasites. The dual serpents, of today's caduceus, were more closely associated with the commercial components of Hermes.

There are no source texts directly attributable to Hippocrates. Rather, writings ascribed to him began to circulate in the century after his death. These writings were gathered into a corpus during the 3rd century CE. The large collection likely had contributors other than Hippocrates. Authors of the Hippocratic corpus divested themselves of the idea that disease was a punishment from the gods, a common belief in ancient Babylonia.

To make the practices more scientific, the new doctrine suggested that illness was the result of meteorological concerns such as seasons and weather. Behaviors were also considered such as diet, exercise, rest and sex. This development of medical doctrine in early Greece oddly paralleled the developments in the late Han Dynasty as they appeared in the *Yellow Emperor's Classic* some 2,000 years ago [7].

Hippocrates, Galen, and Plato promoted humoral views on health and being that influenced the practice of medicine up through the Enlightenment. The initial contemporary practices of medical astrology focused more on nutrition and anatomy. It is the good fortune of the astrological community and those they serve that Project Hindsight and the 'Traditional Revival' brought a renaissance of classical method forward in the contemporary era [9].

METHODS USED FOR THIS BOOK

As a practitioner, my interest is with the integration of premodern, and transcultural thought into contemporary practice.

The inspiration for this work is transdisciplinary at the intersections of astrology and medicine in both early and contemporary thought.[5] These seeds of inspiration germinated at the intersection formed and fed by the confluence of Rudhyarian[6] thought, the cosmologies of Daoism, and premodern Chinese medical thought.

I approach this work from a few points of view. First, a contemplative hermeneutic which applies contemplation to the literature, which leads to insight. I then engage a participatory paradigm where patients participate in the work. Third, I teach the results to students who form a bedrock of reflection and application. The pearls of wisdom derived from this process are presented in a written form for further reflection and refinement.

Gregory Bateson is one of the great thinkers of the 20th century. He argued that the most important task facing us is to learn to think in new ways [10]. Part of new thought is to recapture earlier,

---

[5] Theoretical physicist Basarab Nicolescu provides three axioms of the transdisciplinary method: 1) There are different levels of reality for the Object and the Subject. 2) Resolving paradoxes allows the passage from one level of Reality to another. 3) The structure of Reality is complex: every level is what it is because all the levels exist at the same time.

[6] I am referring to the twentieth-century composer, astrologer, author, Dane Rudhyar.

abandoned methods of thought. My approach to this concern is, again, transdisciplinary. Early and contemporary thought are combined to achieve solutions for the practice of medical astrology that extend beyond the historical methods into the use of cycle-based thinking to develop treatments.

Thus, practice and theory combine as astrology informs the clinical practice, producing, for me, better results than without. The astrological consideration refines clinical judgment, but also creates an opening for deeper dialog between practitioner and client.

In the search for reliable constants, it becomes necessary to seek out a transcultural set of principles that are reliable across multiple points of view. This book focuses especially on astrological methods that transcend the sidereal-tropical conundrum. I do this by focusing upon cycles as tools for knowing, rather than specific divisions of the cycle regarding houses or signs.[7]

LIMITATIONS OF THE BOOK

Only a certain number of perspectives on the cycle can be entertained in this book. My choices are largely predicated on my experience using them in practice. I, therefore focusing on ideas central to astrology, Daoist thought, and alchemy as tools for analyzing the cycle for purposes of developing interventions. This does not preclude the inherent wisdom and power of the views arising from First Nation Peoples, Tibetans, or any other culture which has developed a conception of cycles in relation to the well-being of the individual.

This work is theoretical, as I am not seeking to generate a proof. Rather, I pose principles consistent with the early medical traditions where the use of the 'sign' had mantic or divinatory roots

---

[7]   I do use signs and houses in other areas of my medical astrology practice. This book uses the cycle to provide a foundational point of view.

[11-14]. It is only following the 'Age of Enlightenment' that medicine declined sharply in the use of oracular devices as part of the field of signs.[8]

I reason that the current worldview of Western civilization may be reaching the end of its useful life, primarily due to a shift in how humanity understands and locates itself within the universe.

Humanity has made enormous strides in material welfare and modern conveniences since the beginning of modern science and the Industrial Revolution. However, such progress has come at the cost of ecological devastation, human and social fragmentation, and spiritual impoverishment [15]. Whole systems of thought such as cycle analysis are consistent with thought in premodern cultures, and provide a partial solution to our current plight.

---

[8]   Clinical practice without technology depends upon the sign (that which the practitioner observes) and the symptom (the client's report of experience or symptoms). The process is therefore observational for both the client and the practitioner.

THE CYCLE

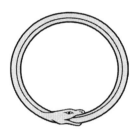

I Hermes, the interpreter of heaven and thrice powerful over earth... The zodiacal circle, which has been born into the limbs and parts and joints proceed out of the cosmos.

—Hermes Trismegistus paraphrased

INTRODUCTION

This chapter introduces the basic concept of the cycle as used in medical astrology. I explore the great circle of the ecliptic as well as diurnal, lunar, and annual movements.

The methods addressed in this book are expanded to the nodal axes of the Moon and can be applied similarly to any planetary nodal axis, or arc of development relative to the cycles of Jupiter, Saturn, and Uranus.

Within the celestial vault moves the wonder of our connection to a vast and mighty cosmos. To bring understanding and meaning, astrologers reduce the sky to the Great Circle of the *ecliptic*. They take the expansive starry Celestial Sphere and collapse it to the pathway of the Sun across the sky, creating the band of the zodiac – the ecliptic – holding the images of life.

Also, there is the *celestial equator*, which projects from the earth's equator into space, and tilts at 23.5° to the ecliptic.

Figure 1

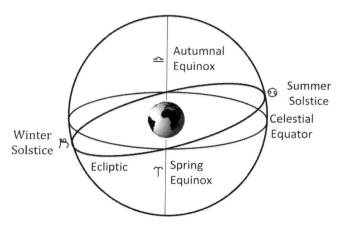

Image of great circles of the celestial equator,
soltices and equinoxes relative to the ecliptic (the 45° band)

One of the prime features of a cycle is increased sensitivity at the angles. The most fundamental Ptolmaic aspects are division by three and two. For the axes, two show up in the opposition at 180^0 whole expanding along dualisms to four, which expresses as the square at 90^0. This is the ground of material experience.

There are other sensitive points in the system besides the Ptolemaic aspects. Planetary stelliums or clusters of planets along the pathway of a cycle can cause distortions in the field as transits are received.

THE 25,800-YEAR PRECESSION OF THE EQUINOXES

The precession of the equinoxes refers to the movement of the first day of spring through the constellations. Also called a Platonic or Great Year, the cycle moves inexorably in opposition to the movement of the planets through the zodiac (See Figures 2,3) [16-18].

Many westerners maintain that Hipparchus discovered the earth's precessional cycle around 130 BC[9]. Astrological practitioners of India, however, likely identified the precession of the equinox some sixteen millennia before Hipparchus (190-120 BCE).

The earliest known mathematical, calendrical and ritual geo-metric texts of India are in the Vedanga, a late adjunct to the development of the Vedic corpus. The astronomical portion was called the Rig Vedanga Jyotisha whose chapters 31-33 explain how to calculate the equinoxes for each year in the five-year yuga cycle, thus providing the first link between the Vedas and the early peak of mathematical astronomy of India in the first millennia BCE [19].

---

[9]   The Zodiac tuning fork is tuned to an octave of this cycle and can be used for matters of the soul's relationship to a grander cosmic time reference. Frequencies as healing agents are addressed in the chapter on Physical Agents and Cycles.

Astrologers of India c. 1800 BCE, used tropical calculations of the solstices and equinoxes as the foundation for their measurement of a year [20]. The mathematics focus upon constellations called Nakshatras. Evidence for this assertion is located in the fifth Rig Vedanga Jyotisha, where it states that a year begins when the Sun is in Shravishtha which is between 23°20′ Capricorn and 6°40′ Aquarius.

The moment of Winter solstice was described as the point when the Sun began moving northward and the days lengthened. These conditions were met approximately 4,000 years ago, providing the evidence for the 1,800 BCE location of the *Rig Vedanga Jyotisha.*

The first day of spring equinox with equal lights will soon occur with the backdrop of the constellation of Aquarius rather than Pisces as the equinox precesses.

The intersection of the *celestial equator* and the *ecliptic* provides the basis for the precession of the equinoxes at the rate of some 1° per 72 years. These intersections are called Vernal points and provide the location of the equinox at zero degrees of the Aries-Libra axis.

The tuning fork called 'Zodiac' resonates with the precession of the equinox and can be tone as a chime or in lower octaves with gongs. See the chapter on physical agents for more details about applying these frequencies.

Figure 2

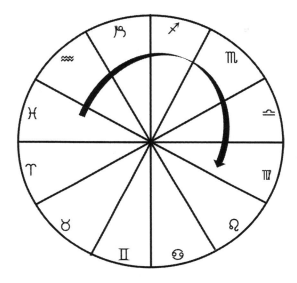

Movement of the equinoctial precession,
also the path of diurnal motion.

THE DIURNAL CYCLE

The daily turning of the planets across the sky have the same apparent clockwise movement as the Great Year. In a 24-hour period, the objects in the sky rotate clockwise, as the observer faces south. Moving from left to right across the sky, planets move through the houses. The diurnal chart analysis is good for analyzing the daily sufferings of life. Stelliums can create stagnation. These planetary locations in the horoscope are hot spots where the various interventions discussed in this book can be applied.

Figure 3

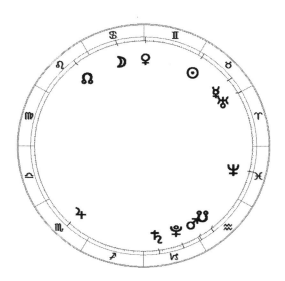

The ascendant is the place on the horizon where the Sun rises. It occurs at the intersection of two great circles, the ecliptic, and horizon. The ascendant provides the beginning point and source of the Zodiac Person's human anatomy, which I will expand in detail later.

ZODIACAL MOTION

Zodiacal motion refers to the movement of planets along the ecliptic and progressively through signs beginning with Aries. This cycle connects deeply with personal destiny and the unfolding of life's purpose. This movement is opposite of motions of the day and the Great Year.

Figure 4

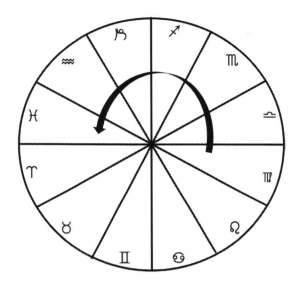

Zodiacal Movement of the planets along the ecliptic

Planets connect with each other in cycles along the path of the ecliptic. These are the pathways of transits and progressions.

THE CIRCLE AND MEANING

Circles are the path of the cycle. This recurrent moment in time is that of the daily, monthly and annual rhythms for the Sun and Moon. All planetary cycles take place within the concept of the circle as it is applied in medical astrology.

Radiant in the glory of life, the native stands upon the earth, facing the southern sky. Daily planetary motions across the sky touch upon the locations where planets are located at the moment of our nativity. This tells of the regular daily occurrences including the highs and lows of energy and symptoms that occur at particular times of day.

The natal chart can be used as a tool for the assessment of daily recurrent health conditions. Say, the client sneezes five times at sunset. I would look first for planets that are angular as the most powerful connection to the moment of sunset.

CIRCLE AND FATE

People project the twelve zodiacal divisions of the ecliptic upon space and assign meaning. Some posit that the chart is subject to free will. This liberated stance comes from a postmodern view of self which is both empowered and isolated. This existential problem becomes a significant feature of our ability to entertain notions of fate and free will.

Take for example, Oedipus and his parents, King Laius and Queen Jocasta. They sought knowledge of the future from the Oracle at Delphi, who informed Jacosta that her son would kill his father and marry his mother. They sent their baby off to the mountains to die. Shepherds saved him and he was adopted by royalty in a nearby country. Oedipus was told the same story by the Oracle at Delphi and left home seeking to avoid his fate. By attempting to control their destiny, all three walked directly into it. I thus maintain that free will is the enactment of fate, just as it was for Oedipus and his parents. Therefore the astrological chart shows that self through which the native expresses true nature.

In medicine, we can posit that fate is realized as people choose their lifestyles.

PEOPLE AND MEDICINE

The great circles are of a singular moment – yet the leaving and return are always at play. Comparable to the beginning, middle and end of any story, the process of emergence from the depths of the void into being and then returning reflects the stirring within all cycles – the *phasis* of mantic arts. The time for self to become revealed or concealed gently stirs from the heart of creation. The evolving nature of the dualisms hot, cold, moist and dry express throughout the days and seasons.

Every planetary orbit forms a dynamic by coming and going. The becoming and returning to the source are implied within diurnal, monthly and annual motions. The planets in the chart sit in relationship to the cycles and affect the flow of enery throughout the cycles.

On a more practical level, cycles are at the root of the comings and goings of life. These cycles are viewed in nested time frames: daily, monthly, yearly larger longer cycles can be related to stages of development such as Jupiter and Saturn cycles. Thus, Jupiter occurs in 12-year, and Saturn occurs in 28-year cycles. The bottom of the cycle takes place at the location of the planet at birth. This idea relies in part upon what is called a synodic cycle: which is the period from one conjunction of two celestial bodies to their next conjunction [21]. Thus, a synod is a place of meeting. These synodic cycles may occur between two planets or a single planet in its relationship to the earth.

Medicinal cycles in the form of therapeutic categories or plant parts resonate with synodic cycles for purposes of enhancing an evolutionary development of the soul. They may also be used remedially for the immediate suffering of the native. An example is to use a medicinal that is downbearing, such as a root for concerns related to a return to source. I will make more therapeutic recommendations in the therapeutic chapters.

Here are complete cycles along the ecliptic for the synodic and sidereal periods of each planet:

Table 1

Planet	Synodic Period (days)	Sidereal Period
Mercury	116	88 days
Venus	584	225 days
Earth	-	1.0 year
Mars	780	1.9 years
Jupiter	399	11.9 years
Saturn	378	29.5 years
Uranus	370	84.0 years
Neptune	368	164.8 years
Pluto	367	248.5 years

Zodiacal Movement of the planets along the ecliptic

My chart tells of the places where I fly and fall, those places where I am free or become stuck. And it is not just for me. Plants have a similar set of cycles, as I am born in concert with all of life. The plant parts relate to portions of the cycle just as the therapeutic categories of herbal medicine affect the cycle in terms of influencing upward and downward, inward and outward motions of the vital life force.

The day, month and year each have a common feature as fundamental cycles. The movement from the appropriate as is the Draconic image with the North Node at the head. Thus, one may use the ascendant as the starting place and take the relationship of the great circle from the location of a birth on the planet.

The nodal axis of the Moon is another point of view which can be especially important in developing treatments that are designed to transform those experiences that can be modified through the exercise of lifestyle changes.

The individual is at the center of many Great Circles. Thus, the ecliptic and the horizon intersect, creating the point where the native's physical presence arrives: the Ascendant. The lunar cycle serves as an archetypal expression for all synodic cycles.

CYCLES IN CLOSING

This chapter on the cycle has focused upon astrological thought tied into the idea of the great circle — that of the ecliptic.

Medical research is rather compelling for a connection between cardiovascular function and lunar cycles [22, 23]. The data on the connectio between the Moon and psychiatric conditions, is however, more tenuous and conflicted [24, 25]. Researchers on both sides of the lunar-psyche connection are likely biased. With some exceptions, sleep studies generally confirm lunar influences [25].

Research on diurnal cycles is often focused on sleep disturbances. Sleep patterns called 'chronotypes' are investigated as a diurnal rhythm [26].

While there is little research on the topic, a symptom arising at a particular time of day points to diurnal rhythms and is suited to chart analysis based on daily motion and a clockwise movement. (An example is a person who gets a headache in the peak of the afternoon with a stellium in the 8th, 9th or 10th houses by nativity, decumbiture or the consultation chart.)

Seasonal allergies and affective disorders take place on an annual basis, so annual rhythms of planetary motion are the place to focus. Obviously, the Sun's aspects are a critical feature of this analysis.

These are a few examples of cycles that can be used on a practical basis for a critical analysis of cosmological conditions in relation to the human experience.

DAOIST CYCLE THOUGHT

...

All things arise in unison.
Thereby we see their return.

All things flourish,
And each returns to its source.

Returning to the source is stillness.
It is returning to one's fate.
Returning to one's fate is eternal.

...

Laozi *Dao De Jing*, Chapter 16

INTRODUCTION TO DAOIST CYCLE THOUGHT

Various cultures have ideas about cycles and their implications for medical practice. I have chosen to elaborate on China's concept of the cycle in relationship to health because material supporting it is developed and available.

The philosophical bases for this medical system are primarily rooted in Daoism,[10] which possesses coherence among philosophy, systematic thought and daily practices.

This chapter provides a view into the cycle from a Daoist perspective. The Daoist concept of the cycle is similar to returning to deep sleep from a waking state through the liminal zone of the dream time and back to source. In the astrological chart, the 4th house cusp connects with deep sleep, the ascendant-descendant axis connects with the liminal zone, and the midheaven with the waking state.

THE WAY

In Daoist thought, *wu ji* denotes a state before time, space and creation. It is the place of all possibilities; and it has no polarity. The *wu ji* splits into *yin* and *yang* while sustaining a state of unity. This process requires *qi,* which pervades the entirety of precosmos and its divisions into *yin* and *yang,* forming the basis of birth and nurture.[11]

---

[10]   Other religio-philosophical traditions affecting the development of Chinese medicine include Confucianism, Buddhism and later Christianity.

[11]   *Yin* is the shady side of the hill. It is lunar cool, shady, moist, and downbearing. *Yang* is the sunny side of the hill. It is solar, warm, dry and upbearing.

Figure 5

Yin and *yang qi* are subsequently divided into the four seasons, bringing forth birth, growth, harvest, and storage [27, p. 34]. After reaching its end, the cycle begins anew. These recursions are without beginning or end. A form of regularity, this cycle limit attractor – or the way of *yin* and *yang* – has no physical appearance or shape. Thus, the way of *yin* and *yang* becomes realized through autopoiesis[12], as self-organizing systems. Further, creation is completed and beings are transformed without end [28, 29].

Cycles are features of the emergence from the Dao and the return. During the emergence, *qi* is vital to the interplay and transformation of *yin* and *yang*. The next evolutionary phase moves through the three treasures of spirit, breath, and essence, which provide a pathway of return to source, moving from the South Node of the Moon to the North Node (See Figure 6). The cosmos presents as the final stage of spontaneous transmutations stemming from original nonbeing into the '10,000 things', which Daoist thought uses as an analogy for all creation.

I associate the South Node with the return to emptiness. This has some resonance with the Indian astrological view of the South Node as a point of liberation and release of the material situation of the native. Whereas the North Node appeals to the desire for acquisition and coming into the world.

---

12   Autopoiesis from Greek αὐτο- (auto-), meaning 'self', and ποίησις (poiesis), meaning 'creation, production'). More details are available in the glossary.

Figure 6

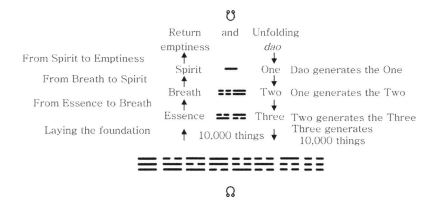

*A variation on Pregadio's representation of
cosmogenesis from the Daode jing [30, p. 55].*

The container of the transformations of cosmogenesis depicted in the image above, has neither shape nor form, and refers to what the Daoists call the 'one cavity.'

In a more inscrutable form, return to emptiness is the root of the void. The sacred is hidden here and appears with the emergence of the original *qi* as one becomes two, two becomes three, and three becomes the 10,000 things.[13] The sacred then disappears when the original qi leaves, returning to emptiness [31]. The mystical, transcendent, and sacred universal phenomena are located within the individual, in the three burning spaces, or 'elixir fields.'[14]

The movement upward transforms from essence to breath to spirit, aligning with the cyclic motion of the planets along the

---

[13] The Daoist cosmological evolution follows on a numerological basis, the bifurcations that take place chaotically within sensitive systems in their evolutionary movement.

[14] The three elixir fields, or Dan Tian can also be called 'energy fields' and have loose correlation with chakras as a three-based system.

zodiac, but also ascending and descending through the three burning spaces. This movement is up the spine and down the front (See Figure 7).

Figure 7

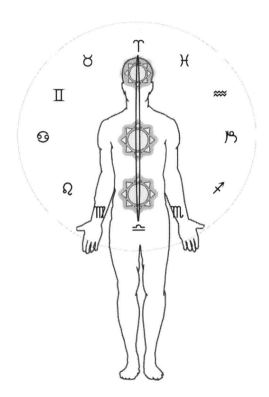

Reduce the zodiac to the center, breathing in up the back and out down the front. If so desired, the return from Libra to Aries moves up the spine and the exit from Aries to Libra down the front.

The planetary movements may be organized into the three spaces where various medical treatments can be delivered. When planets cluster into stelliums at a particular location, treatment strategies may be focused there in order to bring about change related to the archetypal messages contained by the planetary forces.

The question thus becomes: Are we remediating into the presence of the 10,000 things and the matters of the world as the North Node of the Moon, or are we remediating towards the liberation and return to emptiness as in the South Node of the Moon? The answer may be influenced by the stage of development for the individual, whereby the soul evolves into realizing the material or evolves into the return to source. The planetary configurations symbolize the ease or resistance that the client and practitioner will encounter along the way.

DAOIST CYCLE CONCLUSION

The reason I have put this content here is that the cycle has a universal presence and influence on the health of the client. The view from other cultures can enhance the depth of thought and feeling that arises when using the cycle as a tool for care.

The movement from nonbeing into being and the return as described in the diagram derived from Pregadio displays the same set of events taking place in the cycles of astrological concern, including the Saturn cycle, diurnal motion, and zodiacal movement between significant points such as the nodal axis of the Moon. These ideas can be extended to the relationship between planets with beginning, middle, and end. This concept extends to all cyclical phenomena including the movement of the planets against the background of the planetary nodes.

DRACONIC MEDICINE

The Dragon from which all things spring,
One Thing, the formless Dao.

Moving from the unknowable zero point field from which
atomic particles arise, the underlying strings of pure,
wild energy become physical reality.

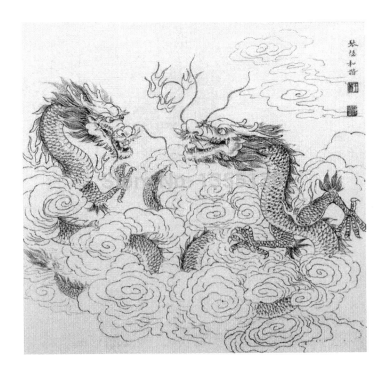

INTRODUCTION TO DRACONIC MEDICINE

Draconic medicine refers to the use of the nodal axis of the Moon for the purpose of developing assessment and treatment plans. The model is flexible and can be applied to herbal and nutritional strategies as well as massage, magnetotherapy, and sound therapies.

As the centerpoint of cycle phenomena, the Dragon has a strong metaphorical correlation with alchemy, appearing in many drawings in European and Chinese alchemical texts. In this chapter, I will provide details on alchemical cycles of transformation as a featured expression of the Dragon.

The question might arise as to why a mythological figure is raised in the context of medical practice. As we have already seen, cycles are critical features of the medical course of care in many traditional cultures. For the purposes of this book, the *Cauda* and *Caput Draconis* are essential features of the cycle phenomena.

BACKGROUND OF THE DRAGON

The Dragon has a significant place throughout the eastern and western cultures. Eastern dragons bestow mystical powers. Western dragons are suggestive of the shroud of illusion surrounding material existence and the desires that make such an existence possible and subsequently necessary.

The Dragon embraces the complex messiness of the light and shadow selves, resolving the paradox. Beyond pleasure, pain, and personal comfort, the universe seeks revolution and resolution as the Dragon eats its own tail.

The word 'dragon' has roots in the Latin term *draconem* or *draco,* the serpent. In Greek, it is *drakon* and generically, *drakontos,* indicating serpent or seafish. Also, sharp-sighted as in drak-, the strong aorist stem of derkesthai "to see clearly," or even literally, "the one with the (deadly) glance." As in martial arts, healing is the right hand path of killing.

THE HEART OF THE DRAGON

Feeling the power of the nodal axis depends in part upon knowing the heart of the Dragon. The Dragon myth exists throughout a range of cultures, taking form in the liminal zones of human experience. Draconic medicine touches upon similar currents expressing through the nodal axis of the Moon.

Before exploring medical applications, I excavate the Dragon from its place in mythic culture, since medicine, culture, and beliefs are inseparable.

CONTEMPORARY ASTROLOGICAL DRAGON DOCTRINE

Much of western astrological doctrine surrounding the Dragon relates the past with the tail and the future with the head. Similarly, the notion of essence and genetic material is tied to the past as far back as the traces of human genomics can be located. Further, it is the aspirations of the mind which direct *qi* into action and lead to the unfolding of future events through the Dragon's head. It is spirit - *the pure light of consciousness which embraces the dark and murky tail of the Dragon, as well as the fire-spewing head of the Dragon* - which creates stability during the transformation and changes of life, as shown by the oscillations of the Moon, Sun and Earth.

The movement along the axis of the Moon takes place either from Dragon's head to tail or from tail to head. Past and future gaze upon each other and the conditions of *becoming* and *returning* merge as the present absorbs the future and allows the past to depart [32].

ALCHEMY – TRANSFORMATION AND THE DRAGON

The Dragon is a central figure in the discipline of alchemy, often used metaphorically to indicate cycles of transformation. As such, this section pertains not only to nodal axes, but also any synodic cycle in its revolutions. These alchemical phases of transformation serve as tools to see a person's location in the cycles of becoming, and to aid in selecting interventions.

Four transformative phases in alchemy include the *nigredo* (blackness), *albedo* (whiteness), *citrinitas* (yellowing), and *rubedo* (redness). The transformative phases of alchemy correspond with the Dragon as follows:

- The *nigredo,* or the dark night of the soul, requires facing the dragon.
- Surrender to the Dragon takes place in the *albedo* stage.
- Becoming the Dragon takes place during the *citrinitas* and *rubedo* phases.

Figure 8

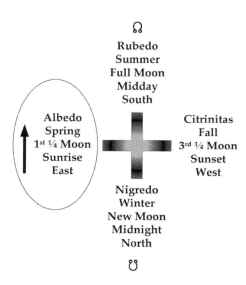

Nigredo is a dark, dense, heavy stage – the moment where that which exists dissolves into the acosmitic zone. This place possesses destructive features leading to sorrowful states. To symbolize this dark moment, alchemists use images such as the black crow, the raven, or the toad (7). The *nigredo* locates at the turning point within the origins of motion: midnight, winter, and the new Moon.

The location of the South Node of the Moon or the 'tail of the Dragon' comports with the origins of all cycles including synods and their conjunction. It serves as the beginning of the cycle within the *nigredo*. The recurrence of cycle origins contain past images associated with critical moments of formation [33]. These moments engender habits derived from social norms and domestication, where the needs and opinions of others affect decisions [34].

The approach to working with the *nigredo* requires searing self-reflection. This reflection focuses upon the shadow self, which is often buried in the unconscious. Bringing such deeply buried material to light can be difficult. One method is to reflect upon agreements made with self and life at the crux of significant events [35].

When facing the Dragon, there is nothing to do but know and accept. Surrender at a primal level tames the Dragon, exalting and liberating consciousness free from judgment.

This act of "Surrendering to the Dragon" brings about the second stage of transformation called the *albedo* or the White Phase. It corresponds with the ascent from the Dragon's tail, through sunrise, spring, or the first quarter of synodic motions.

During the *albedo* stage of purification, the native ceases projection of chaos into the world, instead noticing it within. The *albedo* phase in alchemical drawings is portrayed by a white eagle, dove

23

or swan.[15] *Albedo* associates with silver, the Moon, and embodies as the white virgin. The whitening compares to the coming of dawn after a long night, the moment of rejoicing, hope, and proof that darkness does not last forever.

Citrinitas follows the peak of sunlight as it departs. Still expressing masculine, yang, solar forces, light is brought forward in to the night.[16] The union of male and female takes place as the sun moves below the horizon. This union of day and night it often called the 'chemical wedding.'

From the conjunction of *albedo* and *citrinitas,* philosophical Mercury is born. This phase – *rubedo* – is the triumph of the Work: the creation of the Philosopher's Stone in the form of a transparent red stone, the *summum bonum* and Phoenix of perfect wisdom and happiness. This idea is often expressed in the symbol of the Ouroboros, the Dragon eating its tail.

The head of the Dragon contains the drives, anticipations, and passions towards an unfolding future. The journey requires courage. The tail embraces the depth of past patterns and contains within the potential of liberation.

The ultimate pattern of the Dragon may reveal itself via a final diaspora when it releases its tail from its mouth, and by doing so, frees the inhabitants of all the worlds to return to the domains of nonbeing and essence, a primordeal, precosmic zone.

Surrender to this process of the North and South Nodes of the Moon in which good and bad, positive and negative, health and sickness, life and death, heaven and earth, are poles of existence.

---

[15] As shown in the chart above, the albedo phase relates to the Moon's 1st quarter, spring and sunrise.

[16] The state of *citrinitas* or, 'the yellowing', it is often conflated with the *rubedo* stage by authors after the 15th century.

The universe is not just about personal comfort. Thus, the Dragon embraces the light and shadow selves.

In Daoist alchemy, techniques for unleashing the Dragon center on a practice called the microcosmic orbit. The microcosmic orbit is performed in a deeply relaxed state with the tongue touching the roof of the mouth. Inhaling, the attention is drawn from the coccyx up the spine to the crown of the head. During the exhalation, awareness is drawn from the crown down the central channel on the front of the body all the way through the pelvis to return to the upward movement and inhalation rising along the spine.

Figure 9

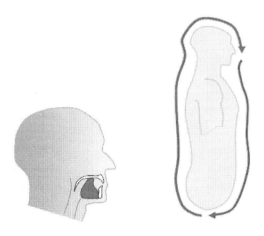

Images modified by author from
Wikimedia Commons, Bostjan46

Disciplines like *Tai Ji* and *Qi Gung* seek to allow the Dragon to live and circulate without interference. Such work allows one to become an effortless and transparent expression of force. This free flow of experience allows movement and clears the stagnations of vitality and blood that presage the array of health conditions.

DRACONIC MEDICINE BACKGROUND

Draconic astrology pertains to the use of the head and tail of the Dragon as the focal point for astrological judgment. The draconic chart, as presented by Pam Crane, assigns 0 degrees Aries to the head of the Dragon rather than the vernal equinox point. The chart sustains the fundamental structure, but the zodiacal placement of the planets change. This derived chart is used for spiritual, soul, and past life assessment [36].

Draconic astrology refers to a zodiacal frame of reference based upon the relationship between the Moon's nodes and Zero Point Aries. Draconic medicine uses the Moon's nodal axis as an alternative Zodiac Person with the North Node at the head and the South Node at the feet. Thus, Draconic medicine employs the dragon as a tool for assessing the native's relationship to past-present-future as a teleological experience of being. Treatments are then developed upon the bases of these time-space considerations.

The nodal axis of the Moon provides an excellent point of departure for medical astrology. This is especially true when no birth time is available. Just as the Sun, Moon, or midday serve as the focus for a chart without a particular time, so also, the North and South node of the Moon.

In draconic medicine, the natal chart is used for matters of constitution and patterns of being. The nativity shows only the potentials, which are a feature of the root self. An example would be the effects of planets squaring the nodal axis. When this happens, there is a chronic-recurrent tendency to use the diaphragm to block feelings that the native seeks to avoid. Over the long term, a constricted diaphragm affects the circulation of blood, lymph, and fluids[17].

---

[17]   Detailed correlations between the Dragon's path and anatomy are addressed in later chapters such as those on physical agents and chakras.

For ease of assessment, we turn the chart so that the head of the Dragon is in the uppermost position. The proximity of planets to various sectors of the dragon can then be easily seen.

The application of the astrological chart to the body is taken from the native's point of view. Thus, the ascendant is on the native's left, descendant on the right, the midheaven is above and the nadir below. With Draconic methods and synods, the South Node - or the beginning of the cycle - is below. This chart orientation then becomes an example of client-centered cosmos and care.

Figure 10

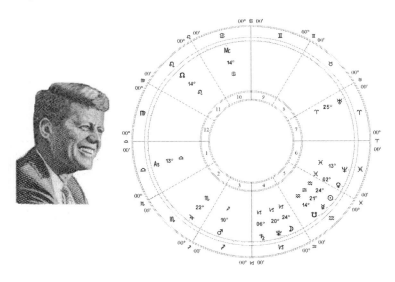

In this figure, President Kennedy faces the chart. The ascending left side of the chart is his left and the descending right is to the right.

The orientation of the chart to the person has its roots in traditions from the bronze age of the Shang[18] and Zhou[19] Dynasties.

---

[18] (ca. 1600–1050 B.C.E.)
[19] (ca. 1046–256 B.C.E.)

Ritual is performed by the Emperor who faces south with the eastern horizon on the left and midheaven above. The perspective is the division of space on the planet from the viewpoint of the pole star. For this reason, the method is absolute for all people, no matter the hemisphere.

This ritual point of view was medicalized in Han Dynasty[20] medical lore. Texts in evidence include the Yellow Emperor's Classic, which forms a portion of state-approved traditional medical programs at both Chinese and international universities [37, 38].

With homage to Bob Jansky as a great medical astrologer, I depart from his Nodal Axis methods. My rationale for placing the chart with the ascendant on the left is a 'client centered' view, whereby the chart is seen through the client's eyes, and not that of the practitioner.

I place the North Node at the 10th house for visual ease. This makes it a more convenient visualization of a whole-body segment than Jansky's method of placing the head to the left at the ascendant and the feet to the right at the descendant.

There is a question as to whether the square to the nodal axis intersects the naval, the diaphragm, or the hara, which is about three finger widths below the naval. When planets square the nodal axis, there is almost always chronic tension in the diaphragm, and this is my most consistent deliberation for the squares to the nodal axis (See Table 2).

---

[20]   (ca. 206 B.C.–220 A.D.)

Table 2

Consideration	Morris	Jansky
Perspective	Ascendant on patient's left (practitioners right)	Ascendant on patient's right (practitioner's left)
Head and tails	North Node at the 10th house cusp	South Node at the ascendant
House system	Whole sign houses	Placidus
Location of the ascendant-descendant axis	Ascendant-Descendant axis intersects the umbilicus	Ascendant-Descendant axis intersects below the umbilicus at the Dan Tian or Kundalini point

In general, I will sustain the head of the human with the head of the Dragon.

Aspirations of the mind direct qi into action leading to future events. Through the pure light of consciousness, the native embraces both the dark and murky tail of the Dragon as well as its fire-spewing head. This embrace of paradox creates stability throughout the transformations and changes of life. Thus, the oscillations of the Moon, Sun, and earth continue.

DRACONIC CONCLUSIONS

Draconic medicine is the practice of using the South and North Nodes of the Moon for assessment and treatment. Rising from the origins, the movement of the Daron from tail to head corresponds with the Daoist concept of returning to the origin as the motion continues past the North Node and returns to the South Node.

CYCLES AND ANATOMY:
HOMO SIGNORUM

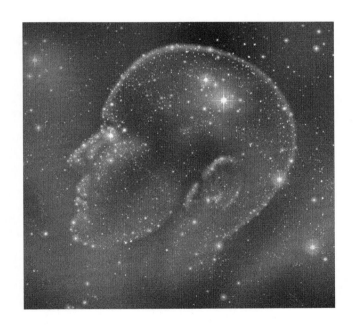

INTRODUCTION TO HOMO SIGNORUM

In this chapter, I will explain the use of anatomical assignments in the traditional astrological sense of signs and houses and their relationship to body parts.

I also expand on the use of these correlations based upon contemporary physics and biological concepts such as fractals and 'whole self-replicating systems'.[21]

The whole-body image may be seen as a microsystem on the hands, feet, scalp, and in fact, any bodily segment. These are holons, replications of the whole in a part, which is also called 'self-replicating systems.' For astrology, these holons are accessed by laying the chart over an area to provide a map which corresponds to the whole body.

Signs and symptoms are presented as the essential matrix from which medical judgment is derived. Further, based upon 40 years of clinical work with 50,000 patients, my clinical judgment and outcomes are better when I include astrology among the clinical signs.

A RATIONALE FOR BODY CORRELATION FRACTALS AND SELF-REPLICATING SYSTEMS

Self-replication is the behavior of a dynamic system that yields identical copies of itself. Cell division is such an example. This idea expands into open systems and can be used to describe the correspondences among the heavens, anatomy, and microsystems of the body.

---

[21]   A whole self-replicating system is a form of biological mirror where a portion of the body is seen as recurrence of another similar portion. Such a concept serves well in treatment.

The fractal is possesses self-similar properties, in that the smaller forms are reduced copies of the larger forms.[22] Examples of the fractal in physiology include the branching pulmonary tracts, intestinal villi, the nervous system, and the vascular system [39, 40]. In plant life, these fractals occur in tree branches and green leaf veins. The self-same and self-organizing systems of new science have resonance with astrology, where various body sections mirror the heavens [39].

Figure 11

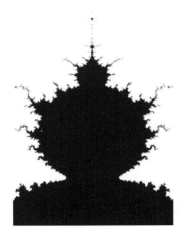

A common pattern created with the Mandelbrot formula.

These fractal phenomena cascade into unlimited holon structures. The influence of these systems on the organism depends on the size of their projections on the surface of body areas such as skin, mucous membranes, and bones.

---

[22]   Benua Mandelbrot brought fractals forward while working in the field of nonlinear equations and complex numbers. His famous Mandelbrot set is used to generate computer graphic images with cascading, self-same images.

Figure 12

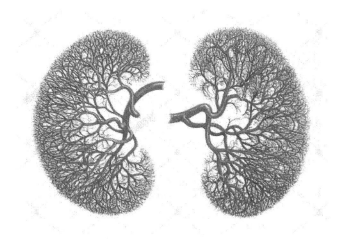

Fractal presentation of the vascular supply to the kidneys.

In nature, seashores replicate from aerial views down to finite detail. They recur in different scales (1:100 m and 1:100 km), yet the patterns are similar.

Holographic and fractal concepts have some resonance with the projection of the sky onto the body, shown when the chart is placed over the body. In this chapter, we will apply the radix chart over the navel (umbilicus), but the turned nodal axis of the Moon can also be placed over body segments such as the leg, back, or arm.

TRADITIONAL ANATOMICAL ASSIGNMENTS

Parts of the body being identified with different spirits and ultimately as the body of the goddess Nut, originated in Egypt and is called *'melothesia.'* These anatomical assignments in astrology are the same for both houses and signs. While traditional astrology in general provides distinct meanings for signs and houses, it is in medical astrology that we may locate the earliest references to the practice of combining sign and house meanings [41].

Table 3

House	Sign	Anatomy
1	Aries	Head
2	Taurus	Throat
3	Gemini	Arms sternum chest
4	Cancer	Chest sides and breast and stomach
5	Leo	Stomach and small intestines
6	Virgo	Umbilical region and pelvis
7	Libra	Kidneys
8	Scorpio	Generative organs, eliminative
9	Sagittarius	Thighs
10	Capricorn	Knees
11	Aquarius	Legs, calves
12	Pisces	Feet

Table Correlations of house, sign, and anatomy

The conception of microcosmos as a mirror of macrocosmos extends throughout the premodern cultures of the Babylonians, Mayans, Egyptians, Hebrews, Chinese, Indians, and the ancient cults of Mithra [41].

During the late Han Dynasty (206 BCE–220 CE), one of the earliest Chinese medical texts called the *Spiritual Axis*, gives the assignment of the planets to organs [42-44] (See Table 4).

Table 4 [45]

Planet	Organ
Mars	Heart
Saturn	Pancreas
Venus	Lungs
Mercury	Kidneys
Jupiter	Liver
Sun	Vitalizes organs
Moon	Containing organs

Planet-organ correspondences from the
Yellow Emperor's Classic [43].

CONTEMPORARY ASTRO-ANATOMY

Dr. William Davidson says that planets rule physiology and signs rule anatomy. The correlation of cosmology, with anatomy, and physiology can vary in a complex world [46]. While Davidson's assignment of planets-to-signs and physiology-to-anatomy can clarify thought, it must be verified through inquiry, rather than take as stone cold fact.

Reinhold Ebertin was a physician astrologer who brought the term 'cosmobiology' into the public light. The method extends upon midpoint astrology as conveyed by Alfred Witte and the Hamburg School [47, 48]. According to Ebertin, the term 'Kosmobiologie' was used by the German medical astrologer Friedrich Feerhow and Swiss statistician Karl Krafft to denote astrological practices that are based upon a foundation of natural sciences [49]. Ebertin defines Cosmobiology as:

> a scientific discipline concerned with the possible correlation between the cosmos and organic life and the effects of cosmic rhythms and stellar motion on man, with all his potentials

and dispositions, his character and the possible turns of fate; it also researches these correlation and effects as mirrored by earth's plant and animal life as a whole. In this endeavor, Cosmobiology utilizes modern-day methods of scientific research, such as statistics, analysis, and computer programming. It is of prime importance, however, in view of the scientific effort expended, not to overlook the macrocosmic and microcosmic interrelations incapable of measurement [49, pp. 8].

Another view upon holism as it applies to medicine is called ECIWO, which is an acronym for 'Embryo Containing Information of the Whole System.' Professor Yingqing Zhang of Shandong University originated the concept [50]. In this model, the whole body is recurring at a 'long bone'. This provides a striking resemblance to the previously discussed fractal structures. Here, the whole body is built as the zodiac on the 2nd metacarpal bone (See Figure 13).

Figure 13

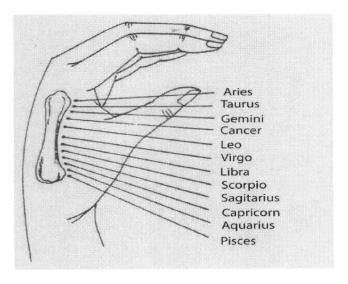

Melothesia on the 2nd metacarpal

Each ECIWO has the potential of the whole in varying degrees and different ways as the organism passes through various stages. The ECIWO phenomena can be seen under favorable conditions, where one single cell has the potential to develop into a new organism, similarly for amputated parts of primitive animals or plants [51].

NODAL AXES AND ANATOMY

The assignment of cosmos to anatomy is a flexible mirroring process. I have presented the zodiac in relationship to body segments. What can be even more effective is the use of the nodal axis of the Moon using 'draconic medicine.'

Draconic medicine assigns the length of the nodal axis to an anatomical segment. In practice, I use the nodal axis as the midline of the body. All the planets in the chart are then collapsed or flattened from their positions directly to the midline, which is the nodal axis of the Moon.

Figure 14

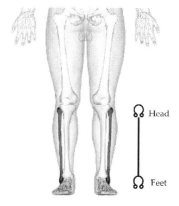

Ω Head

Ω Feet

Thus, any long bone or bodily segment can have an overlay of the nodal axis of the Moon. Collapse the planets around the chart to the nodal axis as a midline in the form of 'dimensional reduction.' To do this, first, turn the chart so that the North Node of the Moon is in the topmost position.

Figure 15

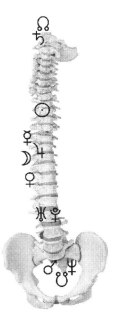

Planets collapse to the midline of the Moon's Nodal Axis
and placed along the spine.

Figure 16

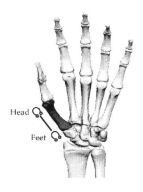

*Example of using any long segment for applying
the Draconic medical method.*

Nodal axis on 1ˢᵗ metacarpal bone.

The practice is not limited to intact long bones, although they
are consistent with ECIWO practices. Consider the application
of acupressure, tuning forks or appropriately diluted essential
oils to the cervical spine.

Figure 17

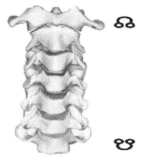

Nodal axis as applied the cervical vertebrae

DISTRIBUTION OF THE CHART TO THE NODAL AXIS

Whole systems mirroring models such as the Moon's nodes or any synodic cycle are not precise. I often divide the body into upper, middle, and lower sectors. The four houses surrounding the North Node are the upper portion of the body. The four houses surrounding the new Ascendant-Descendant axis are the midsection of the torso of the body as a whole. The South Node of the Moon at the new IC,[23] possesses the four houses surrounding it. The planets are then collapsed to the midline in a rough proximity. Precision is achieved by palpation for tender spots or tissue distortions.

Figure 18

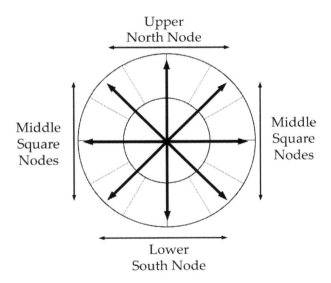

The three burners (Dan Tian) or sectors of the body can be represented along the nodal axis as upper, middle and lower.

---

23   The IC is *Imum Coeli* (Latin for bottom of the sky), it is the opposite of the midheaven.

From the horizon upward and downward by 45⁰ gives a 90⁰ sector for the middle of the body. The middle contains the stomach, pancreas, liver and gallbladder. The sector similarly surrounding the IC provides a view from the pelvis down through the lower limbs. The sector around the MC provides a view to the upper portion of the body including the cardiopulmonary circuit, head, neck and arms.

To say this a little differently, using an equal house system, the South Node becomes the 4th house cusp, and the North Node the 10th house cusp. I then locate the ascendant at the left and the descendant at the right.

From this setup with the North Node at the midheaven, I collapse all the houses aligned directly to the midline. These are wide orbs of influence, and planets may affect adjacent areas.

The 10th and 9th houses correlate with the head and neck. These houses include but are not limited to: eyes, ears, nose and throat, pituitary, thalamus, hypothalamus and the 1st through the 7th cervical vertebrae.

The 11th and 8th houses govern the upper chest, including the heart, lungs, sternum, upper thoracic vertebrae, thymus, structures of the arms, and mediastinum.

The Ascendant-Descendant axis crosses through the diaphragm and may affect everything down to the navel. I palpate this area to confirm planetary effects upon the diaphragm. It will be tense and full just below the rib cage. Openings in the diaphragm allow the esophagus, phrenic and vagus nerves, descending aorta, and inferior vena cava to pass between the thoracic and abdominal cavities. As a result, the diaphragm has systemic effects. Just above the diaphragm and in this sector of the chart are the liver, gallbladder, and pancreas. Thus, the diaphragm is affected by planets squaring the nodal axis.

The 6th-1st houses align with the upper abdomen, this includes the stomach, transverse colon, upper portions of the small intestine and the corresponding aspects of the spine.

The 2nd and 5th houses align with the region between the genitals and knees, while the 3rd and 4th houses align with the feet. The 4th and 3rd houses align with the feet.

SUMMARY OF ASTRO-ANATOMY

The big news is that planets squaring the nodal axis tend to correlate with diaphragmatic tension. The result can be an impact on circulation of blood and fluids throughout the upper middle and lower.

The complexity of fractalating physiological and anatomical conditions allows for the map of the body to be used in many ways.

CHAKRAS AS AN ANATOMICAL VIEW

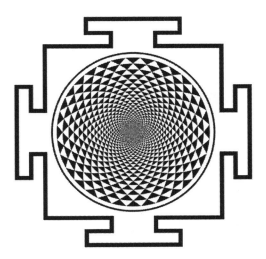

As a tool for organizing anatomical life factors, chakras are known by many and serve as an excellent platform for organizing treatment. Chakras provide an important perspective upon health-care. Serving as neuroendocrinologial nodes, the chakra also describes the physiological and anatomical basis of experience.

The assignment of planets to chakras in this book is based upon the traditions of Ayurveda. Therefore, I rely upon traditional sign rulership. I use outer octave planets, but not for the possession of the mundane features of life on a weekly basis.

The outer octave planets are profoundly impactful when they contact the seven basic planets by transits and progressions. For example, Neptune is often involved in toxic emotional, biological, or chemical exposures. Pluto ties to deep and inexorable changes in the status of tissues. Uranus is often related to shock and trauma or to neurological disturbances.

The seven basic planets ruling the days of the week, also rule the seven chakras in the practice of Ayurveda and Jyotish, the combination of medicine with science of light and the astrology of India.

The Dragon's head and tail align with the rising of kundalini along the spine. Each planet correlates with each chakra in the order of planetary speed, with the slowest at the root chakra. This order is also basically that of the Chaldean order.[24] The exception is that both the Sun and Moon are at the 3rd eye.

---

[24]   Chaldean Order of Planets is Saturn, Jupiter, Mars, Sun, Venus, Mercury, Moon, following the relative order of speed from slowest to fastest.

Figure 19

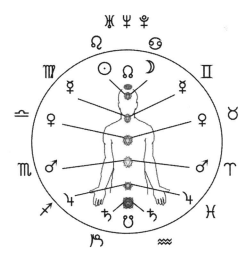

This image shows: a. traditional planetary rulership of signs b. relation-ship of signs and planets to the chakras c. the alignment of the chakras to the nodal axis of the Moon. Uranus, Neptune and Pluto are transpersonal and can interact anywhere by aspect and transit.

Kundalini rises through the awakening chakras. It is the expression of a mystical power, but also the power of sexual union, opening the centers progressively up the spine and releasing through the visionary experience of the 3rd eye. The distinction of opening is rather neutral allowing movement in various directions, while the concept of releasing is a movement away from.

The serpents coiling around the staff of Herme's caduceus share the Indian idea of *ida* and *pingali,* the two sides of the spinal column circulating around the central spinal nerves, or the *shushumna.* On a physical level, these are the central and peripheral nervous systems traveling up and down the spine, supplying organs and serving as the connection between the chakras [52].

These weaving patterns are the warp and woof of the karmic field of endeavor - this in the context of physiology ties directly to the chakra system. I use the Indian astrological methods as having the longest and most substantive consideration of the relationship of the chakras-planets-signs matrix.

The mystical path of the serpent is revealed personally in the axis of the Moon's nodes. The conventional approach to evolutionary astrology gives the future evolution to the North Node of the Moon and the past to the South Node. Indian astrology gives acquisitions and desire to the North Node. This is the incarnating aspect and craves experience through the senses. The Dragon's tail is the area of release, where the material world and the senses fall away.

The chakra system reaches a level of maturity in the literature of the medieval period as displayed through the text, *Sat-Cakra-Nirupana*, written by Purnananda-Svami in 1526 [52]. I use this mini-treatise to form the basis of my thought.

I prefer premodern sources, baked in historical debate, to those of the Theosophical movement vis-à-vis Leadbeater and Besant [53].[25] Thus, I employ the ideas of traditional Indian practices in the form of Jyotish and Ayurveda. I do, however, include the contemporary thought on the endocrine system, based upon anatomical proximity.

Chakras can serve as the focus of treatment, for anatomy and physiology taking place within proximity. This includes organs, tissues, and other structures local to the chakra. They are all relevant to treatment based upon the chakra concept.

The chakras respond well to the herbal class of adaptogens, which modulate the endocrinological-neurological-immunological matrix. Such treatment takes place using what the great sage, Shen Nun, classified as superior herbs. They typically boost qi.

---

[25]   The Theosophical movement has influenced much contemporary discourse on chakras.

I include as adaptogens, herbs that nourish blood, boost vitality, cool and moisten (yin tonics), and enhance metabolic function (yang tonics) [54]. My favorite is the spirit nourishing medicinal *Ganoderma lucidum* (Reishi).

There are many ways to organize thought around energy centers. The Daoists used the idea of the three Dan Tian, upper, middle and lower body as heaven, human and earth respectively. The Kabbalists organize according to the spheres on the tree of life called Sepheroth.

The sephiroth or spheres on the tree of life are presented here with chakras and the three burners, to demonstrate a universality intrinsic to the views of India, Western Mysticism, and Chinese alchemical thought (See Table 5).

The three Dan Tian, or Cinnabar fields, refers to the Chinese medical approach to assigning spiritual and physical significance to the upper, middle, and lower portions of the body. Upper includes everything above the diaphragm. Middle includes the area between the diaphragm and the umbilicus. Lower is everything below the umbilicus (See Table 5).

Table 5

Chakra	Sephiroth	Three Dan Tian
1st root	*Malkuth*	Lower
2nd splenic	*Yesod*	
3rd solar plexus	*Netzach and Hod*	Middle
4th heart	*Tiphareth*	
5th throat	*Da'ath*	Upper
6th third eye	*Chokmah and Binah*	
7th crown	*Kether*	

Following detailed discussion of the chakras in the *Sat-Cakra-Nirupana,* thinking related to the endocrine system was developed between the 17th and 20th centuries [52].

In the table Chakras-Planet-Sound-Gland Correlations, the chakras are associated with sounds. These sounds such as Yam for the heart chakra can be toned for as long as the breath will sustain. As the sound Yam is vibrated, the objective is to have the area around the heart vibrate from the sound. The same is true for each seed syllable as a resonator for each chakra. This activity can have a beneficial impact on the associated endocrine gland.

Table 6

Sanskrit	Chakra	Planetary Ruler	Seed Mantra	Endocrine Gland
Muladhara	1st root	Saturn	Lam	Adrenal
Sadhisthana	2nd splenic	Jupiter	Vam	Gonads
Manipura	3rd solar plexus	Mars	Ram	Pancreas
Anahata	4th heart	Venus	Yam	Thymus
Vishuda	5th throat	Mercury	Ham	Thyroid
Ajna	6th third eye	Sun-Moon	Om	Pineal
Sahasrara	7th crown	Outer Octave Planets		Pituitary

Chakras-Planet-Sound-Gland Correlations

PRACTICAL APPLICATIONS OF THE CHAKRA VIEW

I look at the nodal axis of the Moon and collapse the planets to the axis. Then, if there is a planetary cluster at a particular chakra, I will develop treatments in that area. It could be as simple as laying of hands on an area of the nodal axis where planets are in a stellium.

One approach is to take the tightest-orbed hard aspect between two planets and identify their locations relative to the nodal axis of the Moon. This, then, shows the chakra/s where the most stress is taking place.

I am reminded of a woman who had Uranus and Mercury equally aspecting each other across the throat chakra. She reported thyroid irregularities and injury of the cervical bones due to an accident. This is a common report in my practice.

CHAKRA METHODS

Each planet has an ideal location relative to the chakras. The nodal axis of the Moon serves as the pathway of the kundalini with chakras distributed in to seven locations on the nodal axis. If you observe whether the planet in the chart is in a location consistent with tradition, it will suggest a particular strength in a chakra.

An example is Saturn in the root chakra. There are particular virtues to have a planet in the location where it belongs.

Planetary clusters in a particular chakra will show up in the related life themes. The fundamental energy of a planet will still resonate. Saturn in the heart chakra will make for armoring around the heart and the person must work on feelings of isolation and disconnection. Saturn in the throat chakra can be related to stagnations and obstructions in speech, the thyroid gland or musculoskeletal tissues in the area. The astrological configuration is always confirmed by history and physical examination.

SUMMARY OF HOMO SIGNORUM

The Zodiac Person provides a tool to understand the location of a disease process. The last planet that the Moon contacts suggests the etiology or the source and cause of the condition, while the next planet that the Moon contacts relates to the progress of the condition. These are related to conditions. The signs that are involved tell about the location. The houses have the same representation as signs in medical astrology.

The organization of treatment may be informed by dialog, or on the basis of physical agents, as in the next chapter. Lastly, treatments using the chakras may be organized by the use of herbal medicine.

PHYSICAL AGENTS
AND CYCLES

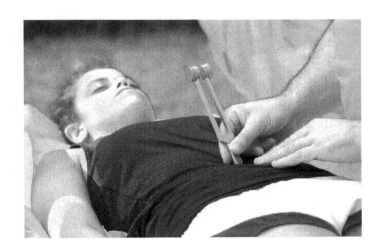

PHYSICAL AGENTS

A physical agent refers to modalities of sound, light, heat, cold, pressure (negative and positive)[26], magnets and water. They are interventions applied to the surface of the body for therapeutic purposes.

Any form of stimulation may be used at the location of a planetary configuration, and which will have systemic effects [55]. [27] In addition to the modalities discussed in the previous paragraph, gem stones, crystals, and essential oils properly diluted and placed over the region can all be used. There are tuning forks tuned to octaves of the average planetary rate of speed. These can be used to stimulate the corresponding body area.

TUNING FORKS

The primary physical agents addressed in this book are tuning forks. This is an agent that astrologers may use intuitively, based upon knowledge and skills related to the domain of astrology.

As the sectors of the chart are placed over the body, then the therapeutic agents that correspond to the planets are placed in their respective positions. Here, we explore the Draconic medical chart for President Kennedy.

---

[26] Positive pressure can be achieved by pushing on an area with a body part or a tool. Negative pressure can be accomplished by cupping the area.

[27] The connective tissue network is an integrated, whole-body system that is amenable to physical manipulation by modalities such as discussed in this chapter. Fascia are composed of an extracellular connective tissue matrix that forms structures surrounding every organ of the body, integrates the musculoskeletal system, and houses the blood and lymphatic vasculature.

Figure 20

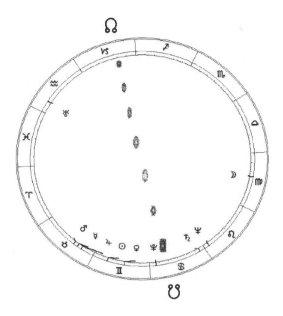

Looking back at President Kennedy's chart, the cluster of planets around the South Node points to the low back. This could also be in the area of the long bones just above the ankles.

GNOSTIC COSMOLOGY AND SOUND HEALING

Cosmology has been addressed as process in the chapter on Daoist Cycles and the chapter related to alchemical processes. These world views address emergence and return of cosmos. Here, I explore cosmology further as a tool for conceptualizing treatment using sound.

Cosmos relates to the state of being. Acosmos is a state of non-being as potential and relates to the potentiality of the *wu ji* as described in Daoist thought. Precosmos supplies a state of anticipation in the movement from the acosmotic towards cosmos and being.

The acosmotic zone has no vibratory state as it exists prior to logos. It is silence preceding particle and wave. Acosmos can be resonated towards becoming through the instability of an evolutionary bifurcation using large un-pitched gongs. I use a 38" Wuhan subatomic gong. It has deep tone with undefined frequencies, raising up into shimmering resonance crossing the liminal zone into a more formed precosmic state.

I use the seven planetary metal Tibetan bowls as a movement towards precosmic potential of the seven planets. They are somewhat dissonant but beginning to have defined pitches, yet with all seven metals they possess the potential for each individual planetary frequency. These have complex wave forms that hold the potential of the seven emanations based upon the planetary orbits. The pitched and spun bowls have pure tone, but do not occupy the transitional space between acosmos and cosmos. It is, rather the complexity of overtones in the Tibetan seven metal hand-hammered bowls that fulfill the precosmotic expression of potential.

Figure 21

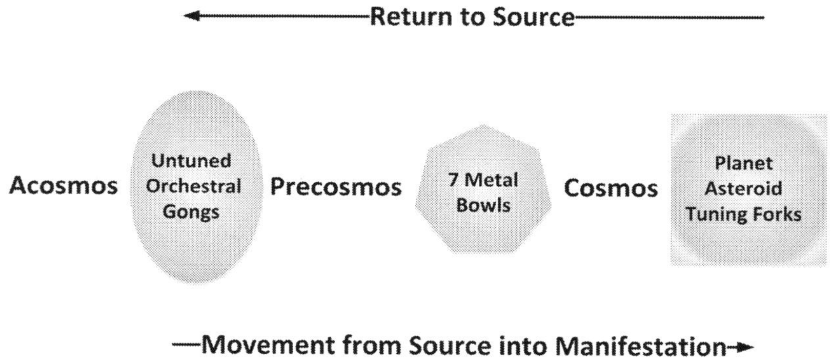

According to Aristotle, the Pythagoreans believed that the planets produced musical notes. His pitches were determined by their velocities and that their velocities were in turn determined by their distances [56]. This worldview is not maintained solely by the Pythagoreans but also the Neoplatonists as can be seen in Plato's *Timeaus* [57, 58].[28] It is not until Kepler's revelation of elliptical orbits, that there is a a crack in the cosmic egg of perfect planetary spherical relations and musical harmony.

Contemporary mathematician/musicologist Hans Custo peers through the crack, leaving the musical worlds of Plato and Pythagorus. Building upon the work of Kepler, Custo sets forth the frequencies for each planet in his book the *Cosmic Octave* [59]. Custo's method takes the mean orbital speed of a celestial object and multiplies it until the frequency can be heard.

For practical application of Custo's work, I use the tuning forks made by Acutonics˚ Institute of Integrative Medicine, which are color coded for easy recognition.

I compare Custo's planet frequency assignments with the equal tempered scale, and the NeoPythagorean, Nichomachus [57]. Each has a place and the NeoPythagorean view of heavier, slower moving planets have lower pitches is quite reasonable.

---

[28]   In the *Timaeus* Plato accounts for the formation of the universe based on order and beauty. This universe is the product of rational, purposive, and beneficent agency in the form of the Demiurge.

Table 7

Spheres of Influence	Custo	Approximation to Equal Temperament	Nichomachus
New Moon	210.42 Hz	G#	E
Full Moon	227.43 Hz	A#	F
Mercury	141.27 Hz	C#	G
Venus	221.23 Hz	A	A
Sun	126.22 HZ	B	*
Mars	144.72 Hz	D	Bb
Jupiter	183.58 Hz	F#	C
Saturn	147.85 Hz	D	D
Uranus	207.36 Hz	G#	*
Neptune	211.44 Hz	G#	*
Pluto	140.25 Hz	C#	*
Eclipse (Saros)	241.56 Hz	B1	*
Zodiac	172.06 HZ	F	E1
Precosmos	Complex overtones and 7 metal Tibetan bowls of antique form		Morris
Acosmos	Large gongs without a tonal center		

Nichomachus' system is consistent with a Platonic world view, where the scale is aligned with perfection throughout the spheres of emanation. In Nichomachus' system, the lower frequencies correlate with slower-moving planets, while higher frequencies correlate with faster-moving planets.

MAGNET THERAPY

Magnets have a long history of therapeutic use, they are noninvasive and generally safe. Magnets can easily be applied according to various ways of mapping the astrological chart to the body. An example is a chart with a stellium surrounding the South Node. The person often has low back pain as did President Kennedy. For treatment, magnets can be placed around the lower back area.

A group of researchers at the Helfgott Research Institute conducted a literature review on magneto therapies. They published in the British Medical Journal's imprint, *Acupuncture in Medicine*. The group culled 50 from 308 studies that met inclusion criteria of: application of permanent magnets on acupoints, case studies, clinical trials, conditions with a medical diagnosis, and publications in Chinese or English. Thirty seven of 42 studies (88%) reported therapeutic benefit. The only adverse events reported were exacerbation of hot flushes and skin irritation from adhesives [60].

TREATMENT BASED UPON THE DRACONIC METHOD

For any physical agent, this method of correlating the nodal axis of the Moon with the body, any whole segment may be used, and it may be reversed. An example is the seven vertebral segments of the neck. The first cervical vertebrae (C1) correlates with the head of the Dragon[29]. This is true for any long bone such as the tibia or any other segment of the body such as the nose or spine.

Any physical agent can be used. Tuning forks are an excellent choice as they can be used by individuals with backgrounds in astrology, and a variety of healing disciplines.

ANATOMICAL APPLICATIONS OF LOCAL SPACE

Local space is an astrological technique for relocation developed by Michael Erlewine [61]. In that method, the practitioner extends the house placements from the location of birth out over the globe.

---

[29]   As with all whole self-replicating systems, the head can mirror the tail of the Dragon.

The application of local space for clinical work is a bit different. In this practice the umbilicus is the focal point, and the chart is placed over the umbilicus. I use the astrological chart as a template to be placed over the body as a form of local space.

Time and movement of the native through time is a different idea. This approach is used to locate stimulation to the body using magnets, pressure, oils, incense, needles, and other materials that affect the person.

The location of the planets is derived by placing the astrological chart over the area of the body to be treated. The ascendant points to the Eastern sector of the body segment, which is the client's left. The midheaven (Medium Coeli [MC]) points to the South, which is the upper portion of the body and relates to the heart. The descendant related to the West, which is the client's right. Lastly, the 4th house cusp (Immum Coeli [IC]) is located in the northern sector of the body and is the pelvis and lower body. [30]

Circular movements of the cosmos have four strata of movement: two are clockwise and two are counterclockwise. Facing south, from the viewpoint of the Pole Star,[31] the diurnal movement of the planets takes place clockwise, while the movement of the planets through the constellations takes place counterclockwise. Similarly, the precession of the equinoxes forming the *great year* takes place clockwise, which is a backward movement through the signs.[32] Superior to this, there is again a counterclockwise movement from a galactic center in clockwise motion and focused down through the constellations into the geocentric location of the practitioner. In application, these concepts are used for applying

---

[30]   The spatial references are ideally based upon the true East point, rather than that which has been modified for the architecture of the treatment space.

[31]   Polaris is the current Pole Star, as it is the closest bright star to the north celestial pole. It is located in the constellation Ursa Minor.

[32]   The movement of the great year is represented in sonic vibration by the Zodiac tuning fork at the frequency of 172.06 Hz.

oils, manipulating fascia with the hands, and the motion of the tuning forks over the body.

Clockwise motions are used to supplement or increase, and counterclockwise motions are used to disperse and reduce. Similarly, Vishnu, Brahma, and Shiva are, respectively, creator, maintainer, and destroyer of worlds, the medical astrologer generates and creates through clockwise motions and returns to acosmos through counterclockwise motions. For the diurnal movement, I use the roots of a plant to get resonance with the bottom of a cycle say, a stellium in the fourth house. More details on this practice in the chapter on herbs.

LOCATION OF TUNING FORKS RELATIVE TO ENERGY SHEATHS

Traditional systems of India consider five energy sheaths, called '*koshas*,' as areas where therapy may be engaged. The seven chakras and five energetic sheaths define a three-dimensional matrix which organizes transpersonal, transcendental, and multidimensional experiences.

Part of the process for locating the conditions of disease includes understanding the location in the body (chakra in this instance), also the location in terms of the energy sheath. Most Vedanta thought places the material body at the outer sheath and the ecstatic, delight-filled states at the interior. I reverse them here, based upon the principle of 'mirrored whole self-replicating systems.'

Figure 22

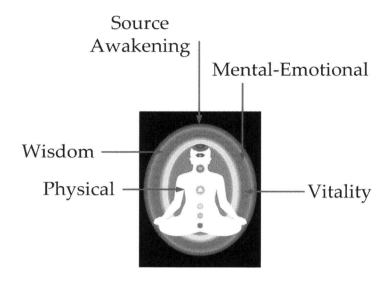

Tuning forks are placed directly upon the body to affect immediate physical conditions and then progressively further from the body until they are pointed away towards the cosmos. I use the latter method when addressing more subtle, spiritual conditions and those relative to distant ancestral currents.

The further into the past along blood lines we see to influence, the further from the body the tuning forks are resonated.

Table 8

Energy Sheath	Element	Needs	General Frequency	Location
Annamaya Kosha (Physical)	Earth, Body	Food	Low frequency tuning forks	Touching body
Pranamaya Kosha (Energy)	Water, Vitality	Air	Low-medium frequency tuning forks	On or close to body
Manomaya Kosha (Mind – Emotions)	Fire, Clarity	Mind	Medium frequency tuning forks	Up to 12" from body
Vijnamaya Kosha (Intellect)	Air, Intuition	Direct Knowledge, Wisdom	Medium-high frequency tuning forks	In the room around the body
Anandamaya Kosha (Source awakening)	Space, Openness	Bliss	High frequency tuning forks	Projected out into space

UMBILICAL METHOD AND THE HOROSCOPE

The center of the astrological chart symbolizes the place on earth where the native takes their first breath. The umbilicus is the center of the native with the same correspondence to the center of the cosmos as the earth in a geocentric universe.

The umbilicus connects us to our birth. It is the point of separation at the time of the cutting, and this original scar is with us the rest of our lives. It is the umbilicus where the geometric patterns formed by the relationships of the planets to each other focus light into the body. The umbilical method provides access to the portal created by the first scar a person experiences at birth.

The circle around the perimeter of the umbilicus aligns with the ecliptic and therefore, the location of the planets. The umbilicus provides the intersection between the MC-IC axis and the Ascendant-Descendent axis.[33] The ascendant is located to the client's left while the midheaven is upward from the umbilicus. The angles formed by the major Ptolomeic aspects tend to create congestive patterns that can be palpated as tender knots in the tissues around the umbilicus.

SPECIFIC UMBILICUS TREATMENT

Treatment of the umbilicus can be performed by stimulating select planetary locations as deemed significant by the astrologer. Any number of materials may be used including: essential oils in an appropriate base, fingers, magnets, crystals, and tuning forks.

Take for instance, a hard aspect between Saturn in the 1st house, and Pluto in the 10th house. This configuration may be invoked by stimulating towards the root of the navel from the left side midpoint of the navel. As the person faces south, the left midpoint of the navel corresponds with the ascendant.

---

[33] It is important to note that the perspective of the chart is that of the client and not the practitioner. Thus, the midheaven is the upper body, the ascendant is the client's left, the descendent is the client's right, and the Immum Coeli is the client's lower body.

Figure 23

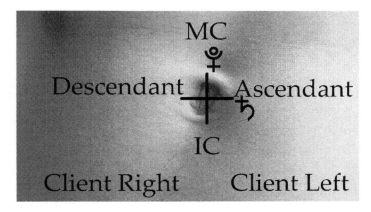

There are tuning forks that are tuned to each of the primary planets, Sun, Moon, and the outer octave planets of Uranus, Neptune, and Pluto. Acutonics' has also provided tuning forks in low, medium, and high octaves at the planetary frequencies of Chiron, Sedna, and Nibiru. They have also provided high-pitched tuning forks aligned to the frequencies of asteroid goddesses Vesta, Juno, Ceres, and Pallas Athena. The vibratory frequencies of dwarf planet Sedna, bring up the archetypal influences, and provide an opportunity to resolve deep acosmic and concerns, existential crises of being which can lead to deep depressions. Hypervigilance, anxiety, and fear related to cataclysmic phenomena in the world resonate with the forces of Nibiru.

HOT AND COLD APPLICATIONS

Fire warms and may be applied in the form of incense or moxibustion.[34] If Mars and the Moon are conspiring to cause inflammation and swelling, ice can be used. The hands must be warmed to

---

[34] Moxibustion is the use of mugwort specially prepared for direct or indirect application to an area in order to generate warmth, increase circulation, and stimulate organ function. Ethical considerations require that a practitioner have training in a procedure prior to its use.

palpate cold tissues. Cold planets such as Saturn are often present with cold tissues – a perfect scenario for a warming strategy. An infrared lamp is wonderful on a cold lower back that is being influenced by Saturn. A washrag soaked in hot water is particularly effective as well.

My favorite way to alternate hot and cold is to go back and for between hot earth and cold water in the summer, in my bare feet. This stimulates circulatory function at a deep level.

Color and Light Therapies

I have worn the color of the planet which rules the day of the week for 28 years. It has become a fluid practice, whereby different traditions cross-over, and the ruling planet becomes a decent substitute when I have neglected the laundry. Wearing the color of the planet/day is a very common practice in Ayurveda.[35] There are differing points of view regarding color assignments to the planets. Most of these are culturally bound. Table – gives a comparison of the uses in Ayurveda, Renaissance and Medieval concerns. I also place my own point of view.

There are some color therapeutic devices on the market. I invite you to explore, but will make no recommendations here. There are also color therapeutic practices that use color gel slides, projectors, and other very simple means of saturating a room with light. The colored gels can also be placed over the tissues that are affected.

For the practices I am sharing here, a focalized light pen with changeable filters is the best solution. That way if one were seeking to stimulate Saturn at its location around the umbilicus it would be very easily accomplished.

---

[35]   This is the humorally based traditional medicine of India.

Table 9

Planet	Morris	Lad[36]	Lilly [62]	Al Biruni [63, 64]
Sun Sunday	orange, yellow, red	gold, red, orange, yellow	yellow red purple	Reddish, yellow[37]
Moon Monday	white	white	green orange yellow white	blue orange yellow
Mercury Wednesday	green, variegated colors	green	blue grey mixed	blue grey pink yellow
Venus Friday	pink and floral patterns	purple, bright colors	light blue light green white	white yellow
Mars Tuesday	Red	Red orange	Red	Red
Jupiter Thursday	purple	yellow	green	dust, brown white, yellow, glittering
Saturn Saturday	blue, black	blue, black, dark colors	white, pale ashy black dark	black, mixed with yellow dark
Uranus	dazzling[38]			
Neptune	iridescent			
Pluto	ultraviolet, violet			

---

[36] Dr. Vasant Lad is a leading teacher of Ayurveda in the West. I have seen him practice the daily wearing of colors represented here.

[37] Al Biruni also gives the color of the planet ruling the planetary hour on the Sun's day.

[38] The Uranus, Neptune, and Pluto colors are from Elbert Benjamine.

SUMMARY OF PHYSICAL AGENTS

This chapter focused on some therapeutics that can be applied to the surface of the body. I have paid particular attention to the use of tuning forks. I believe that if an astrologer can get involved with a procedure related to the practice of astrology such as applying tuning forks to the surface of the body, that they can then build a more regular interaction clientele and achieve greater depth than that which can be gained in less frequent encounters.

CONSTITUTION, CYCLES AND HUMORS

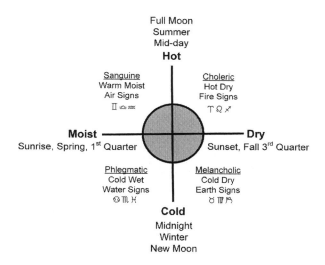

Full Moon
Summer
Mid-day
Hot

Sanguine
Warm Moist
Air Signs
♊ ♎ ♒

Choleric
Hot Dry
Fire Signs
♈ ♌ ♐

Moist ——————— **Dry**
Sunrise, Spring, 1ˢᵗ Quarter   Sunset, Fall 3ʳᵈ Quarter

Phlegmatic
Cold Wet
Water Signs
♋ ♏ ♓

Melancholic
Cold Dry
Earth Signs
♉ ♍ ♑

Cold
Midnight
Winter
New Moon

A composite image of the humoral relations
in the day-month-year view

Rooted in the essence of the ancestors. Blood flows from generation
to generation. The importance of building treatments that take
into consideration the family of origin heighten.

INTRODUCTION TO CYCLES AND CONSTITUTION

The humors as medical thought were lost following the Age of Enlightenment. They have been sustained in the practice of Chinese medicine, Southern Folk Medicine,[39] and Ayurveda [65]. There is, fortunately, a resurgence of traditional humoral-based medical thought where medical astrology can provide some of its best service.

This chapter focuses on the cycle in relationship to the constitution, which is often called the temperament [8, 66]. The methods can be seen in a mature form within the Renaissance stylings of Culpeper and Lilly [67-71].

There are several forms of the constitution: 1) the nature of the individual, 2) the stage of development (babies have a phlegmatic constitution, whereas the elderly tend towards a cold, dry, melancholic state), and 3) acquired constitution as in a shock causing the hair to grow grey. In addition to the humoral constructs of Galen, there are also ways to describe constitution as organs (a big heart). In this chapter, the discussion focuses on the nature of the individual.

The condition of the day, month, and year form a cornerstone in the methods of evaluation. Although planetary influences on the ascendant can skew the patterns shown by the cycles, but factors, even the smallest, must receive due consideration in the development of interventions. An example of this would be a person born in the summer, during the full Moon at midday, who should be of a hot constitution. If the ascendant is conjunct

---

[39] Southern folk medicine is a tradition of medicine that survived the economic forces of industrialized medicine in poor states such as Alabama. The corporatized chemical-surgical beliefs had insufficient economic incentive to pursue the Alabama marketplace. The medicine there was a Creole combination of early Greek humoral medicine rooted in the thinking of Galen and the local indigenous knowledge of medicinal plants.

Saturn, a cold planet, then cold will also be clearly visible in the conditions of the native.

CONSTITUTION AS PRINCIPLE

Most pre-enlightenment medical cultures assess the constitution. These include China, Africa, India, indigenous and first nation communities, Unani, Tibb, and southern folk medicine of North America. In the astrology, of Medieval, and Renaissance Europe, the constitution is called temperament [8, 72, 73]. [40] [41]

The constitution relates to the essential nature of being. It refers to the physical vitality, health, and strength. It can also be used to describe a person's mental or psychological makeup. One aspect of the constitution can be built as the unique expression of that part of consciousness occurring as a thread of awareness of 'I' over time. "Whereas space is central to the world of objects, time is central to the world of self" [74, p. 150].

Thomas Sydenham, a famous 17th Century English physician, expanded the idea constitution to include a complex set of natural events, including quality of soil, climate, seasons, rain, drought, and centers of pestilence and famine. He suggests that constitution revolves around a hidden mystery. Such constitutions rarely have symptoms, nor are they defined by symptoms [75, 76]. An astrological chart is a tool for seeing into this hidden mystery.

For constitution, I speak to the continuity of being from the beginning of life. In addition to a continuous presence, stages of development, and acquired conditions imprint upon the terrain.

---

[40] Lee Lehman's work on Traditional Medial Astrology stands as the authoritative address upon method.

[41] Sirius software has a module designed to employ Dr. Lehman's excavation of traditional medical astrology methods. In Sirius, go: Listing, Ancient Western, 1 refranation etc.

The terrain into which the individual incarnates becomes a part of self. Thus, the 'ground of being' arises within the ebb and flow of the daily-monthly-annual cycles bringing the fundamental background of the constitution as a process of individuation.

CONSTITUTIONAL ANALYSIS

Analyzing the constitution requires assessing the humors attendant upon the constitution. The diagnosis of the humors from a medical astrology point of view best includes a complete history and physical examination so that all expressions of temperament receive due consideration.

Outlier data are important. When a person with strong evidence of fire and moisture has signs of cold, it must all be accounted for, even if it is not clinically obvious. We are into a world of complexity, where the subtle gains relevance. It is similar to the 'butterfly effect', whereby the butterfly, which flaps its wings in Tokyo, causes a tornado in Connecticut. This can be referred to as 'minute first causes.'

The analysis of constitution evolves first and foremost from the condition of the ascendant as it is representative of the body. Planets located close to the ascendant will impart their humoral influences upon the constitution according to their nature. The sign rising at the moment of birth will also impart its influences.

The planet ruling the sign which rises over the ascendant will impart its nature, but most importantly, the humoral quality of the sign where the ascendant ruler is placed has the strongest influence.[42] For instance, if Scorpio is rising and Mars is placed in a fire sign, the constitution will be hot. If, however, Mars is placed in a water sign, the constitution will have cold and

---

[42] There is a special consideration called the *Almuten* which is dealt with under dignities whereby a planet other than the ruler gains primacy in its dominion over a sign and consequently a house or domicile.

wet influences. The picture becomes more complicated if, say, Saturn, a cold, dry planet, is close to the ascendant at the same time that the ruler of the ascendant is in a water sign. There is then the influence of cold and dry, combined with cold and wet. Of one thing we can be certain, the person will have tendencies towards coldness.

The condition of the ascendant tends to dominate the constitutional status of individual. The influences of the monthly, daily, and annual cycles tend to be more of a constant pastel background to the sharp relief of the influences that directly act on the ascendant.

SEASON

A background influence is tied to the seasons. For summer births, place a check in the hot box. The winter-born tend to be colder, and the spring-birthed people have a slight damp influence, while the autumnal folks have a dry influence (See Figure 24).

Figure 24

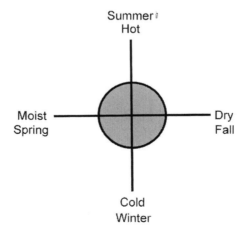

The seasons in relationship to constitution

MOON SIGN AND PHASE

An idea of the cycle possessing eight phases can be seen in cultures such as Africa, early China, and Native American. Rudhyar also suggests a plant cycle to the 8-fold division of the Moon's cycle. Rudhyar's approach to evaluating the status of the Moon regarding phases may be applied to any cycle [77]. This is an extension on the four-fold divisions that are used throughout this book.

The simpler four phase division of a cycle, for the Moon, begins with the new Moon and progresses to the first quarter on its way to the full Moon. Then the retreat begins through the third quarter and back to the new Moon.

The cycles of the Moon are nested in the time frame of the year, with the new Moon as winter, first quarter as spring, the full Moon as summer and the last quarter having resonance with autumn.

The Moon's motions in its cycle is a zodiacal and moves counterclockwise in a monthly rhythm. The diurnal motion of the sensitive points is clockwise. This daily motion is nested within the cycle of the Moon as a smaller time frame. As such, the conditions of the smaller time frame take place within the context of the influences governing the larger time frame.

Table 10 [43]

Phase	Days	Degrees	Cycle	Plant Part	Treatment Principle
New Moon	Dark to 3 ½ days after the New Moon	0-45°	Birth	Gemma Sprouts	Boost Qi and Yang, Warm
Crescent Moon	3 ½ to 7 days after the New Moon	45-90°	Emerge	Shoots	Upbearing[44]
First Quarter Moon	7 to 10 1/2 days after the New Moon	90-135°	Growth	Bark	Regulate qi and up-bear
Gibbous Moon	10 1/2 to 15 days after the New Moon	135-180°	Expand	Branches Leaves	Disperse and open surface
Full Moon Phase	15 to 18 ½ days after the New Moon	180-225°	Peak	Flowers, Fruits	Clear, Cool, open
Disseminating Gibbous Moon	3 ½ to 7 days after the Full Moon	225-270°	Scatter	Nuts, Seeds	Descend qi, moisten, purge
Third Quarter Moon	7 to 10 ½ days after the Full Moon	270-315°	Let go	Bark	Downbearing drain, diurese
Balsamic/ Dark Moon	10 ½ days after the Full Moon to the New Moon	315-360°	Retreat	Roots	Moisten and Blood

---

[43] Adaptation of Rudhyar's Moon cycle concept. I suspect this may have been influenced by Rudolph Steiner's thoughts on plant life.

[44] Upbearing refers to the general tendency that a medicinal has to bring about a movement of the vital life force upward. Similarly for downward.

The tides provide direct evidence of the Moon's influence upon bodies of water – and since we are mostly water, the Moon could have a significant impact on humanity. It is the Moon which can be used as a general principle in building and draining techniques. The waxing Moon is an excellent time to begin tonic and nourishing therapies. The waning Moon is a good time for starting purges, cleanses and other draining techniques, such as diuresis, bleeding and clearing heat toxins (See Figure 25).

Figure 25

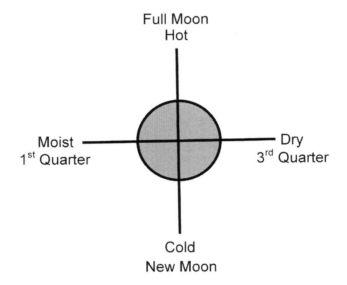

The humoral features of the Moon's cycle

The Moon is one of the most important considerations in medical astrology, or any of the mantic disciplines for that matter. Planets that aspect the Moon should be considered, particularly if they are strong, such as a bodily conjunction.

LOCATION OF THE SUN IN THE SKY

Location of Sun in the sky sets up the background.

Figure 26

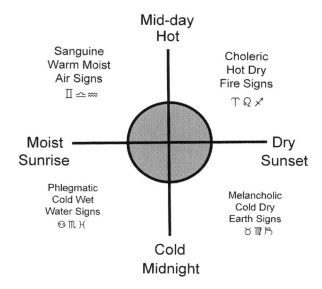

Diurnal motion and humors

The daily motion of light waxing and waning provides a backdrop for the real with respect to immediate cosmological and meteorological factors in horary practice. But, in this view, we consider the birth chart, and the moment of birth in the day becomes one pastel color in the presentation of a whole complicated person.

CONDITION OF ASCENDANT

Planets very close to or in conjunction with the ascendant will affect the body condition. The planet which rules the sign upon the ascendant also affects the body, but also the sign in which that ruler is placed has influence. Further, the planets which gaze upon the ascendant will affect the constitution and the nature of the body.

CYCLES AND THE ASSESSMENT OF CONSTITUTION

The cycle is one of the most fundamental features of existence and consequently of human experience. The assessment of constitution presented here is one derived from practices from the Medieval and Renaissance eras. The application of the day-month-year cycles transcends the bounds of the tropical and sidereal zodiacs, relying upon the cyclical nature of these time frames. Each contributes to a pastel-like background upon which the condition of the ascendant is given primacy - not just the ascendant, but rather the humoral condition of the sign in which the ruler of the ascendant is placed.

The practice of medicine includes the observation of both signs and symptoms. The signs are those objective or subjective events observed by the practitioner. The symptoms are the shared experiences of the client. The value of astrology is not located within an absolute and provable truth. Rather, we are looking for the ebb and flow of a living, moving, and breathing body which has complexity and changeability at its core.

Table shows the relationship of the cycles to the humors as a single unit. For the day, sunrise is counted as moist, midday as hot, sunset as dry and midnight as cold. Similarly, the Moon cycle and the seasonal cycle all provide a mosaic.

Table 11

Humors and their Features – adapted from Lilly [71]						
Quality	Element	Humor		Seat	Discharge	Planet
Moist and Warm	Air	Sanguine	Blood	Liver	Blood	Jupiter: warming
Dry and Hot	Fire	Choleric	Yellow Bile	Gall Bladder	Urine	Mars: drying
Wet and Cold[45]	Water	Phlegmatic	Phlegm	Lungs	Phlegm	Venus: moistening
Dry and Cold	Earth	Melancholic	Black Bile	Spleen	Stool	Saturn: cooling
Mercury takes on the attributes of the sign and plane with which he associates						

While cycles are significant features of the constitution, knowledge of the humoral tendencies of the planets is also necessary. Here is a brief set of correlations for the planetary influences.

Sun:

Sun aligns with the up-bearing portion of the cycle. He is choleric, hot, dry, the most powerful fire, and goodness. Sun influences the heart, vitality, and general warming metabolic function. Sun resonates in the sympathetic nervous system response range, stimulating survival responses. Pathologies of Sun include fatigue, ailments of heart and upper spinal region, fevers and breaking down of tissues, organic ailments, and fainting spells.

---

45   Here, we can see the controversy over the warm-cold nature of Venus in the lore.

Moon:

Moon aligns with a downbearing portion of the cycle. She is phlegmatic, cold, and moist, embracing good and evil. Women's reproductive cycle is also under the influence of Moon. She is second only to Sun for influence over the general health and vitality. Moon is important for the stomach and linings of various tissues. Moon resonates in the parasympathetic response range, around feeding and breeding. Her pathologies include atonicity and edema. Being sedative and soporific, she can be a factor in mental complaints. Moon governs diseases of the stomach and all contained spaces.

Mercury:

Being Mercurial, the motions of the cycle are enhanced in any direction. Mercury takes up the influences of planets he associates with. Mercury is of his own accord, not hot, moist, cold, nor dry. Mercury governs conscious thoughts, the brain, nervous system, the frequency of the electromagnetic vibrations of the body, breath, perception, and biocommunication. The pathologies of Mercury relate to nervousness, mental agitation, neuralgia, neuritis, sciatica, hay fever, asthma, and some dermatological and intestinal complaints.

Venus:

Venus as evening star gently guides energy downward in the cycle. When she appears as the morning star she has an upbearing quality. She is sanguine/phlegmatic and cold or warm depending upon whether it is a morning star (cold) or an evening star (warm). Venus rules the kidneys, venous blood, and the veins, skin, and hair. She influences endocrine secretions related to sexuality and parasympathetic responses. Her pathologies include endocrine conditions, especially the thyroid and reproductive organs. Venus governs acne that is hormonally centered, such as the rash that breaks out at puberty or just before the menses, and female complaints. Venus can be lax and remissive.

Mars:

Mar's impact on the cycle is to generally up-bear vital life force. He is choleric, hot, and dry. He rules the muscular system, immune system, red corpuscles, and hemoglobin. His influence reaches the bladder, gonads, and the secretion of both adrenalin and cortin by the adrenal glands. He often presents with the sympathetic nervous system response of fight or flight. Mars pathologies include inflammation, burning sensations, good fiery skin conditions, acute disease, and pain.

Jupiter:

Jupiter can ease the pathway, with a tendency towards upbearing and downbearing. He is sanguine, soft, moist, hot; lord of blood which is moist and hot. Moist factors pull energy downward, while warmth is upbearing. The pathologies of Jupiter arrive as accumulations and overabundance, since the person can be corpulent. Jupiter is associated with acidosis, diabetes, biliousness, catarrh, autointoxication, carbuncles, neoplasias, and fatty tumors. Jupiter is also associated with a parasympathetic state of feed or breed.

Saturn:

Saturn is downbearing in term of the cold, dry gives a slight upbearing, and this comes as focus. He is melancholic, hard, dry, cold. He leads to the formation of support tissues, influencing the joints, bones, ligaments, teeth, and mineral salts of the body. His pathologies are restrictions and binding, depletion, and obstructions.

TRANSPERSONAL PLANETS

Uranus:

Uranus sends energy upward and associates with kundalini awakening. Uranus is cold. There can be sudden electrical changes in the nervous system, such as an alternation of the electrical purkinje fibers that operate heart rhythms. He is a sympathetic nervous system stimulator. His pathologies include accidents, strokes, and sudden health events. The lasting impact often affects the nervous system in general or at the level of local motor and sensory function.

Neptune:

Neptune diffuses and descends energy. Neptune loosens the integrity of membranes. Consistent with general malaise, there can also be seeping exposure to chemicals, psychism, spirit afflictions, and toxins. Neptune increases the influence of the parasympathetic nervous system.

Pluto:

Pluto connects with deep, inexorable, cataclysmic change. Genetics and epigenetics are part of Pluto's story as he usually stimulates the sympathetic nervous system and can switch to parasympathic amplification.

CLINICAL PRESENTATION OF THE HUMORS

The idea of the humors in this instance is not literal; rather, they are an abstraction. The practitioner assigns meaning to the observed signs and symptoms that are interpreted as hot, cold, moist, and dry. It is important to note at this moment that all scientific endeavor involves abstraction, whether quantitative or qualitative. The humors are a quintessential feature of qualitative organization of the observed signs and symptoms in the clinic.

Astrology provides enlargement on conventional medical workups. That is, astrology expands on the normal history and physical with laboratory-based blood workups and imaging such as X-rays, and it must be taken into account along with standard clinical observations.

The match or mismatch of signs often speaks to prognosis. The more inconsistent the observed 'signs and symptoms,' the poorer the prognosis. The reason for this is that coherence is consistent with healthy physiological function. The chaos suggested by disparate signs and symptoms is suggestive of a lower capacity for recovery.

COLD CONDITION

Signs of cold must be seen to name the phlegmatic and melancholic constitutions. The person feels chilled. Cold produces clear fluids without odor. The urine is pale, the sputum on the tongue is clear with clear bubbles. The bowel movement can be watery with no odor. The skin around the elbows and knees may be cold to the touch. This is different from cold hands and feet which may be cold due to stress and vasoconstriction.

Muscles are soft and fleshy. Client is quiet and withdrawn with preference for warm food and drink.

They dress warmly and like heat. The metabolism is slow and there is little thirst. A cold client is often tired, sleeps a lot, and has a tendency to feel depressed, quiet and withdrawn. Their health is worse in cold weather.

FOODS FOR COLD CONDITIONS

Regular, warming aerobic exercise is critical for improving general metabolic warmth. Therapeutic foods include warm lamb or beef dishes, dark poultry, meat-based soups and stews, free-range eggs, eel, trout, and wild salmon. Beneficial vegetables include cooked root veggies, baked winter squash, onions, and mustard greens. Nuts and seeds are warming, as are butter, cinnamon, garlic, ginger, turmeric, and pepper. Helpful grains include oatmeal, quinoa, and buckwheat. Food and drinks should be cooked and consumed warm. Minimize salads, raw fruits, frozen desserts, pasta, white flour, and iced beverages.

HOT CONDITION

Look for signs and symptoms of both the choleric and sanguine constitutions. Choleric is dry and sanguine moist, but they are both warm. When full-on heat is present, there will be redness, fluids will darken and thicken, and odor will increase. The tongue is red, the eyes can be red or injected. The skin is red. The urine is dark and yellow. The phlegm turns thick and is yellow or green.

The client is ruddy with a tendency to feel warm and is uncomfortable in hot weather; therefore, he or she dresses in short sleeves. The urine can be dark with an odor. The client may suffer fever blisters, canker sores, constipation, headaches, bleeding, and high blood pressure. Such people are often thirsty, craving cold drinks. There is a tendency to be talkative, critical, impatient, irritable, or angry, and sleep is often restless, with disturbing dreams.

In addition to a constitutional state, heat patterns may be due to overwork, alcohol, sugar, hot weather, stress, or spicy and greasy foods.

FOODS FOR HOT CONDITIONS

Ideal foods are salads, cucumbers, and lightly cooked green leafy vegetables, especially spinach and watercress. Vegetables of all kinds are helpful, whereas meats should be limited. Other cooling foods include melons, pears, bean dishes, mung beans, sprouts, sushi, non-spicy soups, and ample water. Mint is a beneficial cooling herb, and it is wise to reduce pepper, garlic, ginger, and onions.

DRY CONDITION

Dry signs and symptoms are necessary in the choleric and melancholic temperaments. Dry people feel dry to the touch. The tongue appears dry.[46] The pulse may float, and it is distinct from the surrounding ground substance. The fluid output is often scanty and that includes menstruation. There should be a good deal of thirst. The cheeks may be gaunt and slightly concave, as the tissues there are not filled with fluids.

There may be dandruff, dry stool, constipation, preference for warm liquids in small sips, and dry throat or eyes. Fluid excretions from the body are reduced. Dryness in seniors presents with visible blood vessels on the top of the hands.

A dry pattern is a deficiency of yin or fluids. Hormones, skin oils, saliva, digestive juices and secretions provide us our yin element. Fluids are akin to a car's antifreeze; when low you can easily overheat or freeze. We see dryness at menopause, or as we age and skin becomes dry. Although hot flashes feel like heat, they are a sign of diminishing yin, which allows the normal heat of the body to go unchecked. Stress also depletes yin.

FOODS FOR DRY CONDITIONS

Beneficial fats are critical. Healthful choices include fatty fish, free-range eggs, grass-fed butter, goat and sheep cheeses, olive and coconut oil, dark poultry meat, pork, nuts, and avocado. Soups and stews rich with grass-fed animal fats are very helpful. Other moistening foods include black beans, green beans, Napa cabbage, winter squash, yams, sea vegetables, millet, whole wheat, fermented soy, and shellfish.

---

[46] When I see a dry tongue, I ask if there is thirst. If there is no thirst with a dry tongue, the complexity is increased and greater care is recommended.

DAMP CONDITION

Wet constitutional features are palpable. One can squeeze the forearm and feel the congested fluids. If the fluids are hot, they have color and odor; if they are cold, they have no odor and are clear. The wet constitution is consistent with phlegmatic when cold and with sanguine when hot. The face will be somewhat plump and on the red side for the sanguine and on the pale side for the phlegmatic constitution. Further wet features may be a thick or wide tongue, wetness on the surface, or sputum stringing between the teeth and the tongue. The pulse may be deep.

These clients have a strong dislike of humidity, as health declines when exposed to damp. They may have a stuffy nose, postnasal drip, and mental fogginess. There can be abdominal bloating, retention of fluids, and little thirst or hunger. The person can be overweight, and soft. The urine tends to be cloudy. The eyes or face can be puffy; the client can feel easily short of breath, with a feeling of heaviness especially in lower body.

FOODS FOR DAMP CONDITIONS

Dampness can be associated with cold or heat and is exacerbated by damp living conditions. Chronic dampness is brought on by eating on the run, excessive worry, or from a diet rich in fried foods, breads, pasta, commercial dairy, ice cream, and other sweets. Too many salads and raw fruits weaken digestion and lead to dampness. Aerobic exercise is essential for balance.

Helpful foods include lightly cooked greens, including broccoli, turnip greens, asparagus, and kale. Fish and grilled or roasted meats and poultry are balancing. The best grains for a damp pattern are rye and jasmine, and basmati rice, as well as sprouted grains. Radishes, turnips, pumpkin seeds, green tea, and bitter foods and herbs help to dry dampness. Sweets, dairy, and starchy foods contribute to dampness. Ice cream, lasagna, white bread, and milk should be avoided.

CLEANSES

Cleanses are often best conducted during the spring season, as the energy is moving upward and outward. Winter not as helpful as the energy is moving down and inward. This is contrary to the use of the Moon cycle, where the waning Moon is more useful for elimination and giving blood. In general, it is better to cleanse as the energy moves outwards rather than to cleanse in the fall and winter, as the natural inclination is for energies to withdraw and go inward.

When treating along these cycles we are always faced with the decision between sympathy and antipathy. Shall I oppose the warmth of summer or go with it? A common practice in the Fire Spirit school of Chengdu in the Sichuan Province is to use hot herbs such as properly prepared aconite (which is a poisonous plant) along with cinnamon cooked with lamb. This solstice remedy anticipates the return to the darkest and coldest portion of the cycle in winter.

HERBAL APPROACHES
TO THE CYCLE

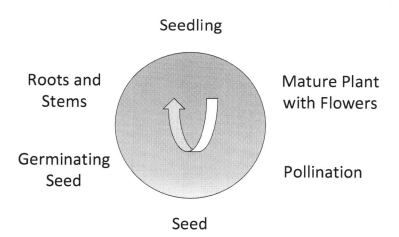

Seedling

Roots and
Stems

Mature Plant
with Flowers

Germinating
Seed

Pollination

Seed

INTRODUCTION TO THE CYCLE IN HERBAL MEDICINE

This chapter is focused upon the selection of medicinals based upon their capacity to initiate and affect transformation throughout the cycles by increasing or reducing movement. It builds on the relationship between 'the way a native moves through time and cosmos' in relation to the plant and mineral kingdoms.

The astrological chart shows the location of planets as points in space. These points suggest the places where vitality stagnates or quickens in its movement. Plant medicine can be targeted to transform these nodes of stagnation and quickening in the cycle.

I analyze the chart in a clockwise fashion in order to address the concerns of daily life. Herbal strategies of upbearing and downbearing are applied to the areas where a planetary stellium is suggestive of stagnation. Attention is also given to those areas where the energy may quicken, such as Mars in Aries in the upper left quadrant. In this situation I may use cooling and moistening foods or herbs to slow down the hot, dry nature of Mars.

Herbal formulas written for the purpose of the soul's evolution and growth move counterclockwise, following the zodiacal path of movement. The planetary humors block or facilitate the movement of life force, according to location and the humoral nature of the planet.

The principles of treatment are the same whether diurnal or zodiacal in motion. The focus of upbearing and downbearing will change, though. That cluster of planets around the ascendant which must be raised in the daily concerns related to diurnal motion must be descended in the longer-term concerns of evolutionary growth through the zodiacal motion of the planets over time.

Annual, monthly and daily motions form the backdrop of the constitution and the humoral state. These are the most fundamental cycles.

The archetypal forces of each planet evolve through its orbital. Thus, Saturn's cycle weaves with the adulting process in relationship with Jupiter as two social planets that show the relationship between the native and their ecopsychosocial[47] circumstances. Venus, of course, seeks the gentle loving touch and the same for the other senses on the path to beauty. Mercury seeks the mind, while Mars seeks to act.

CYCLE INTERVENTIONS WITH HERBS

The source of this method rests with Chinese medical thought about how transformation takes place on a cyclical basis. This form of herbalism derives of an ecopsychosocial world view similar to that of Han Dynasty (c. 200 CE) medical practitioners. It was one where existential,[48] social, locational, meteorological, dietary, and constitutional factors were part of consideration for health.

One example is a Han Dynasty practitioner who considered cosmos in the course of care. Seasons and the diurnal motions of the Sun through the houses, were often a part of the health assessment. The movement of the Sun through the houses on a daily basis matched the organ clock and the movement of qi through the meridian systems of acupuncture. The meridian concept will be addressed in another book.

---

47 Ecopsychosocial is a reference to the internal-external ecosystems in terms of cosmos, the spiritual and material components of being as intra - and intersubjective experiences.

48 Existentialism is thought to originate with Kierkegaard. I classify it as the crisis of being human. As such, this is a concern for all ages and times.

THE CYCLE FOR PSYCHOSOCIAL CONCERNS

Plant life operates in lock step with seasonal, diurnal and lunar influences. Just as the plants experience a complex ecopsychosocial state, so do our clients who consume these plants as medicine.

As a reiteration, zodiacal motion of the planets appears counterclockwise when the native faces south. The zodiacal motion emphasizes individual's relationship to a greater cosmic whole.

Diurnal planetary movements appear to move clockwise and relate to the concerns of daily life. These two perspectives sustain in the southern hemisphere, as the prospect of revolution is seen from the viewpoint of Polaris, the pole star, gazing upon a spinning planet.

Here are some considerations for cycle-based herbal treatments for existential crises, with anxiety and depression related to the problem of being. If the presenting complaint is a concern of daily existence, I explore the nativity in clockwise fashion.

If the energy is sinking and depressed, I look for sensitive planetary conditions rising on the left.[49] Treatment is focused on herbs that direct the energy upward - that is, they upbear the vital life forces.[50] If it is a hot planet such as Mars, I will use a cooling diaphoretic (upbearing) herb, such as mint. If it is cold, I will use a warming upbearing medicinal such as ginger or cinnamon, or twigs and leaves and suchlike.

If there is anxiety, I look toward the descending portion of the cycle for clues to treatment. I am searching for herbal solutions that interact with the descending portion of the cycle, bringing the vital life forces down and inward. This might be addressed as simply as recommending roots.

---

[49]   Say, Mars in the 1st house square Saturn in the 4th house.
[50]   See appendix 1 for medicinal categories and their effects on upward and downward motion.

THE HERBS

The ideas in this section are a synthesis of contemporary thought upon plant consciousness, extraction of the thought expressed by biologist-chemist-Waldorf teacher, Ernst Michael Kranich (1929-2007), who was influenced heavily by Rudolph Steiner and Johann Wolfgang von Goethe [78].

This view, stimulated by Kranich et al., is an appreciation of the archetypal plant. Such a view embraces form and function. These processes are extensions into the environment and not operating as isolated molecular structures, chemical interactions or genetics.

The plant points beyond the boundaries of its form (Saturn). As part of its environment, it is rooted in soil, absorbing moisture (lower part of the cycle). Through the leaves, it maintains a relationship and exchange with the substances of the atmosphere (Mercury). From the earth it receives the forces necessary for life growth and formation [78].

Humans, heaven and earth, are conceptualized as a three-fold expression of reality in Chinese medicine. Just as the plant, humans, heaven and earth are composed of upward and downward bearing forces. Extending this thought into the existential realm, the upward and downward forces open and close the realms of objective and subjective experience.

In the view of Steiner, the growing portion of the plant corresponds with particular planetary forces [78, 79]. The original image as archetype holds within a higher order of both sensation and feeling.

Plant life with upward growing shoots has a relationship with Sun's yang forces. The shoot extends upward, radiantly establishing a direction of growth, unfolding with the increasing light of day. In contrast, root development and growth correspond to Moon's field effect, composed of yin forces. The roots reach into the earth, towards darkness, moisture, and nourishment from the soil.

Taking the thought of Goethe et al., the beginning of the cycle originates with that which becomes the plant, sprouting from the seed [80]. Vital force, as Wilhelm Reich and Chinese medicine would see it, possesses the boundary of protective energy. Here, the influence of the Sun resonates with features of the plant which radiate upward and outward. Similarly, Moon's forces press inward and downward, connecting, and supplementing the nutritive aspects of life.[51]

Upward, radiating processes bring about the blossom. It is here that the forces of Venus interact with those of Sun. The flavors spicy and sweet resonate with Sun and Venus, bringing them closer.

Mercury in expression and form operates as a place of communication in leaves, where there is an exchange with the atmosphere of ionic and carbon-based materials. The winding nature of the vine is a place where the interaction of Mercury and Sun take place.

Mars and Sun interactions can be seen in plants that are biennial, with two-year cycles. The Martian-Solar influences are spicy and upbearing and can be easily seen in plants such as members of the onion family, mullein, parsley, fennel, carrot, and some hollyhocks.

Jupiter and Saturn influences are seen in annual rings of large trees. Barks, resins, twigs and leaves allow for the ability to taste the medicine internally. Forest therapy is the best way to gain the blessings and healings of the old ones.

---

51   A good example of herbs that emphasize this polarized Sol-Lunar influence in a clinical setting are cinnamon twigs (*Ramulus Cinnamomum verum* – Sun) and white peony rootlets (*Rhizoma Peonia lactiflora*). Cinnamon opens the surface and peony nourishes and softens, closing to the interior.

THE SUN AND THE CENTER SHOOT

The central shoot of a plant around which the other features of the plant revolve, serves as center of the plant, possessing a morphic resonance with the Sun as center of the solar system. The shoot also connects with the origins of the cycles within the alchemical negredo. It pushes upward and outward, reaching from the darkest part of the cycle towards the light.[52]

The connection of shoots to the Sun becomes apparent during the spring and summer seasons where 'heliotropic activity' follows the pathway of the Sun across the sky.

During daytime the Sun empowers the morphogenetic field of the plant to take shape. The central shoot emerges different in time periods according to genus and species as the season progresses from spring, to midsummer. For instance, in the northern hemisphere, buttercup, geranium, and lily shoots reach full development in May.

Emergence of the shoot upward, pushes from the depths of night, and the depth of winter. It reaches upward into the cycle towards that of spring – transforming cold into moisture.

DOCTRINE OF SIGNATURES

The ability for a plant to affect motion in a cycle can be seen in part through the doctrine of signatures. This type of thinking can be associated with the doctrine, which was abandoned in the wake of scientism for the proof of single agent mechanistic causation.

Father of pharmacy Dioscorides, and the medical researcher of antiquity, Galen, discuss the doctrine of signatures. The doctrine suggests that herbs resembling various parts of the body, can be

---

52   There is a botanical treatment method that uses shoots and sprouts as tools for nourishing and detoxification. It is called 'gemmotherapy.'

used to treat ailments of those body parts. 'Nature marks each growth ... according to its curative benefit,' Paracelsus agrees (1493–1541) [1]. Jacob Böhme first presented the term 'doctrine of signatures' in his 1621 book *The Signature of All Things* [1].

In this book, the doctrine of signatures is a suggestive feature, rather than a concern of certainty. The doctrine is a heuristic, which is a tool for thinking.

Rather than reproducible constants serving to arbitrate truth, the doctrine of signatures deserves to be returned to its rightful place in the noosphere. The doctrine may enjoy the practical uses that it held for indigenous cultures.

The use of science to dismiss the doctrine of signatures is no different from science as a tool of empire, which is addressed by physicist Vandana Shiva:

> Dominant scientific knowledge thus breeds a monoculture of the mind by making space for local alternatives to disappear, very much like monocultures of introduced plant varieties leading to the displacement and destruction of local diversity. ... By elevating itself above society and other knowledge systems from the domain of reliable and systematic knowledge, the dominant system creates its exclusive monopoly [81, p12].

Returning to the doctrine and away from the reasons for its castigation, plant resins (read: blood), have a resonance with human blood. Indeed, frankincense and myrrh are plant resins that move blood. Colors are a clue - for instance, hawthorne berry is red and affects the heart and circulation.

Plant parts, colors, flavors, and location of the plant community are all features which can be applied according to the doctrine of signatures. Not only the chemical features such as the bioflavonoids, but the plant morphology, taste, color, and location have an aggregate impact upon the native's experience, especially in the recursions of life experiences.

While the tendencies within the doctrine are not composed of predictable and repeatable reliability, they serve a deeper understanding. The practitioner must have a relationship with the plant material to make the recommendation.

The ability to recall its taste is foremost among the various relationships one can have with a medicinal plant. More importantly, I draw upon indigenous knowledge whereby the plant initiates the practitioner and empowers this individual in the use of the medicine. This process requires regular use of plant material, the study of transcultural lore regarding the medicines, and a relationship with the plant in its location through the seasons. Sometimes there is a song that rises. For me, there is a dialog in spirit.

HERBAL PRESCRIBING BY HOROSCOPE

Herbal prescribing works differently from that of physical medicine, where anatomy connects with the chart images. Rather, the herbal approach deals with functional features of medicinal classifications. The alchemical *conjunctio* takes place at the synodic node at the bottom of the cycle, which is equivalent to the beginning (See Figure 27).

Figure 27

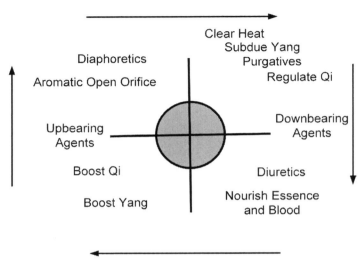

Cycles and Medicinal Categories

Figure 27 provides suggestions regarding the effect of medic-inal classifications upon a client and as represented in a great circle. When planets cluster together, recurrent difficulties and stagnations occur in the life of the native relative to the planets involved, their placement, and the houses they possess. Planets in hard aspect also contribute. But never underestimate the power of a harmonious aspect to create stagnation, when two planets encourage one another to hang back and maintain the status quo. The most important feature is the feeling of the planets involved.

Agents that boost vitality tend to have an upward arc of motion, just as diaphoretics which cause sweat and peripheral vasodilation have an upward movement. Purgatives, diuretics, and carminatives tend to bear downward. This up and down movement creates the potential for emerging from the depths of the night into the sunrise and following the path of the Sun through the day.

The doctrine of signatures may be employed to understand the relationship between plant life and the comings and goings of the cosmos. It is, however, important to note that the doctrine is not one of certainty and absolute reproducibility, but rather, that of tendency. Thus, roots bring us to the beginning of the cycle, while the bark xylem and phloem transport nutrients from the roots to the upper portions of the plant as its circulatory system.

Figure 28

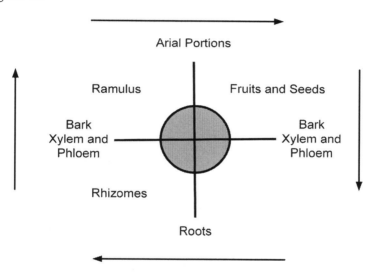

Plant Parts and the Cycle

Plant parts have a resonance with the cycles of movement as well. The correspondences between planets and material objects have been recorded by many over the millennia and there are many sources with extensive tables of correspondences. Table -- shows plant to planet correlations used by Henry Cornelius Agrippa (See Table 12).

Table 12

Planet	Plant
Jupiter	Fruit bearing
Venus	Flower-bearing
Mercury	Seeds and Bark
Saturn	Roots
Mars	Wood
Moon	Leaves

In Agrippa's view, Saturn and Jupiter are related to fruiting plants, but not those that flower. Venus and Mercury affiliate with plants that flower, and seed, but not those that bear fruit. Plant life that reproduce of their own accord without seed are of the Moon and Saturn [82]. Examples include budding succulents such as aloes, spores for ferns and shoots for potatoes.

The evolutionary status of the emotional state can be seen in the cycle of the Moon. Hard aspects to the Moon during the first quarter can be addressed with barks, twigs, and flowers which lead the vitality up and out past the difficult moment of the emerging Moon. These materials are vasodilatory and open to the surface. If, however, the native has difficulty retreating to spend time in deeper reflective stances, then the descending and grounding function of roots may be employed as an influence. Contrary to popular opinion, good-quality ginseng assists this process as it 'returns to source.'

The doctrine of correspondences should not replace knowledge of the specific actions for a particular medicinal herb. The obligation is on the practitioner to know the indications and contraindications for medicinals. For instance, since ginseng can cause sodium retention, it is contraindicated in high blood pressure. So is licorice.

Figure 29

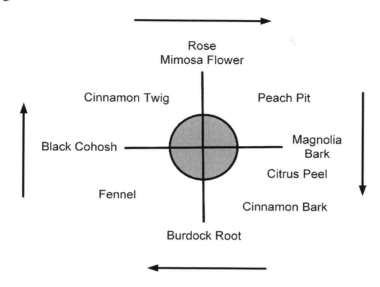

Examples of Plants and Movement

On a daily basis, we experience the entirety of the astrological chart as the Sun in its diurnal motion passes through each house. Keep a daily journal which tracks the movement of the Sun and Moon through each portion of the chart and the places where the difficulties and stagnations, as well as the victories and triumphs, become evident. This practice can be illuminating in combination with chart analysis and the selection of a plant ally which resonates with the sensitive points within a cycle.

FLAVOR FACTORS

Flavor varies in strength, and has the ability to affect the eco-psychosocial conditions of the client. The power of taste can be used to focus on a particular portion of the cycle.

A small amount of a strong taste can override that which is weaker. Bitter Mars overrides all other tastes, and salty nullifies all other tastes. Therefore, small amounts are in order, but be ever mindful that it is easy to make a nasty-tasting herb formula and can be difficult to make a tasty formula.

Sweet, Venus, operates as a vehicle for other tastes. It not only makes other herbs more palatable but enhances uptake of the medicinal at the cellular level via sugar pathways. The spicy, Jupiterian liver flavor enhances the uptake of other medicinals by vasodilation, therefore enhancing absorption of medicinals through the intestinal tract, and also into local tissues.

One may employ the meanings of the planets in the context of cycles. The archetypal experience is part of the process. Or the planets may be viewed functionally in relationship to time, expressing as stagnation[53] and accumulation. The planets then point to locations in the cycle where the energy must be quickened or slowed. One client had a red, inflamed upper back. The consulation chart showed Mars and Sun conjunct in the upper third of the Moon's nodal axis. The treatment concept was to cool and downbear the energy. Roots of green plants do this.

---

[53] Stress and lack of movement both cause stagnation. Over time, stagnation can accumulate as palpable material, an accumulation such as food stagnation.

Table 13

Flavors associated with the planets adapted from William Lilly [83]			Plant Examples
Saturn	Bitter-astringent	Sour and sharp and astringent	Oak
Venus	Sweet	Pleasant smell, sweet flavor as from oils and fats	Seeds
Mars	Bitter-pungent	Sharp caustic and burning, slightly harsh	Gentiana
Jupiter	Delectable	Rich and sweet: moist, creamy, and unctuous	Dates
Mercury	Mixed	A combination of flavors that are quickening, subtle and penetrating	Citrus peel
Moon	Watery	A watery or slightly sweet taste, but overall bland	Lily bulb
Venus	Spicy	Aromatic flavors, pungent,	Cinnamon

Flavors, when organized from strongest to weakest are: bitter, salty, pungent, sour, astringent and sweet. This idea can affect how much of an herb is placed into a formula.

HEAVY & LIGHT PROPERTIES OF TASTE

Flavors move up and down. The lighter flavors tend to lift through the cycle, while the heavier flavors generate a return to the source. This point of view is a good way to organize the directional pull of an herb without memorization. Moving from lightest, to heaviest, they go: bitter, pungent, sour, astringent, salty, sweet

HEATING & COOLING EFFECT OF TASTE

Warmer medicinals tend to have a rising effect, while cooler agents can direct the vital life force downward, influencing the cycles of life throughout the nested time frames from day to month, year, and multiyear cycles. From hot to cold, in general: pungent, sour, salty, sweet, astringent, bitter. I use bitter flavors when a client has heat above in the body, which should also be demonstrated astrologically.

MOISTENING & DRYING EFFECTS OF TASTE

The moister a medicinal is, the more downbearing capacity it has for 'returning to source.' The dryer the medicinal, the more power to uplift through the cycles of life. In order, moist to dry: sweet, salty, sour, astringent, bitter, pungent. The dryer flavors correspond with the planets, Saturn, Mars, and Sun. The moister flavors relate with Moon, Venus, and Jupiter. Mercury goes either way, depending on the surrounding conditions.

For instance, a consultation chart has Saturn in the 7th house, the person standing on earth, will have cold and dry in the middle (head to MC, feet to IC). A moistening agent will assist descent of qi to source. Since Saturn is also cold, warming can be of assistance. Cinnamon bark is warming, moistening and downbearing.

TASTE IN EXCESS & DEFICIENCY

Too much of a taste can damage the humor it aggravates. Extremes can even damage the humor that a flavor benefits. Deficiency of a taste will first damage the humor it benefits, and then the humor it aggravates. Too much of any taste will damage the body as a whole, not just the associated humor, tissue, or organ.

As an example, too much salty flavor over time, can affect the circulatory system, and therefore, circulation in general.

BALANCE & TASTE

Opposite tastes tend to neutralize each other. More importantly, it allows one to act on the basis of continua such as:

Table 14

Up	Down
Bitter is Light	Sweet is Heavy
Pungent Expands	Astringent Contracts

Other opposites such as sweet/sour can be used to balance or amplify herbal actions.[54]

PUNGENT

The pungent taste has a dispersing action. It opens upward and outward affecting the cycle accordingly. The expansive feature of the pungent flavor connects with Jupiter.

Pungency opens the lungs and pores of the skin. The action takes place due to the volatile oils present in plants with a pungent/spicy flavor. These oils irritate the tissues, causing an expulsion through the skin and lungs. This influence increases the free exchange of substances from inside to outside. Psychologically, it frees up the human tendency towards grasping for states of consciousness as well as items of comfort or security. The action of the pungent flavor opens a person to exchange.

The basic properties of the pungent flavor are light hot and dry, moving the synodic cycle out from the source at the beginning of the cycle. This pungent nature tends to be catabolic, drying, and absorptive. It produces a tingling sensation on the tongue and can increase salivation. These effects of the pungent flavor are primarily due to the content of essential oils.

---

[54] The sweet-sour axis can be applied to the axis of softening and condensing. Sweet builds and softens, while sour condenses. Further, a small portion of the opposite flavor can enhance the direction and action of its opposite.

Sometimes called spicy, the pungent flavor has a warming effect which increases the internal fire. It also reduces spasm of smooth muscle, relieving congestion. Clinically it is used for respiratory problems such as a cough, colds, and asthma; it is also used for digestive, heart, and skin problems. Obesity, parasites, diabetes, loss of appetite, and dental pain have all been treated with materials containing this flavor.

Pungency is used to treat what Chinese doctors call qi stagnation, which can include: fullness, distension, and/or pain.

Cautions for using the pungent flavor incude: dryness, yin deficiency (hyperthyroidism), and scattered thoughts. Excessive pungent flavor can cause fainting, debility, impotence, giddiness, burning sensations, dry cough, tremors, thirst, and nerve pain.

The pungent flavor is found among the following therapies: culinary, interior warming, diaphoretics, analgesics, dry damp, and, dissolve phlegm. Typical sources of pungency are ginger, cayenne, cardamon, and mint.

SALTY

The salty flavor relates to water, the sea of which we are composed. It dissolves downward through the synodic cycle.

The organ associated with the salty flavor is the kidney, which regulates blood salt content and is assigned to the lower section of the body in Chinese medicine. Salty flavors calm the nerves and relieve anxiety. Salt changes the consistency of saliva, causes a burning sensation in the mouth, softens food, and puts an edge on the appetite. Its properties are heavy, solvent, and wet; it can be hot or cool depending on the salt. In small doses, it acts as a purgative or laxative; in large doses it acts as an emetic. The salty flavor moistens the intestines and softens accumulations, assisting in the breakdown of tissues (catabolism). Salty flavors cleanse the body's channels.

The salty flavor is used to treat weight problems, bumps, cysts, tumors, lymph congestion, loss of appetite, expelling wind, and to relieve constipation, phlegm accumulations, and difficult to expectorate phlegm.

Excessive salt intake can result in thirst, loss of consciousness, fever, eczema, erysipelas, gastritis, dropsy, impairment of sense organs, high blood pressure, loose teeth, hair graying or loss, and a host of other symptoms characterized by excessive heat and dampness. The tendency of salt to attract fluids results in a physical sensation of laxness. Salt is contraindicated for gastritis, high blood pressure, skin complaints, fluid swelling, and hemorrhages.

The salty taste is used for therapies such as purging, emesis, aphrodisiac, digestive issues, anticancer, and weight loss.

Sources of the salty taste are sea vegetables, sea shells, sea salt, rock salt, and animal remedies.[55]

BITTER

Bitter is the most powerful flavor and the most avoided in the American diet. It can blot out other flavors. In small doses, bitter flavor opens upward and outward in synodic motion. In large doses it drains heat downward through the cycle.

Bitter connects with ether, creating spaciousness. The etheric connection allows the bitter flavor to penetrate the finest channels of energy. Its basic properties are light, cold, and dry. It reduces fire and water and promotes wind, clearing the psyche, it increases lightness of mind. This effect on clearing the mind is why the Chinese associate the bitter flavor with the heart.

---

[55] Animal remedies can include materials from bovine or porcine tissues such as the kidneys, thyroid, and pancreas. They can also include insects such as cicadas and ants.

Bitter dries damp and disperses. It is also used to cleanse the blood, detoxify, and clear heat. The bitter flavor is used to treat insufficient stomach acid, fever, obesity, diabetes, skin diseases, poor appetite, gastritis, jaundice, and increased secretions.

Excessive intake of bitter can lead to raw mucosa and ducts, physical weakness, dejection, sleepiness, vertigo, harming of the upright qi, and degeneration.

Contraindications for bitter are deficient cold problems, and lowered sperm count.

Sources of the bitter flavor are Oregon grape root, gentian, and dandelion.

SOUR

The sour taste guides downward in synodic cycles. It relates to the liver, and gallbladder. Organic acids are what generate this flavor. It awakens the mind and senses. Typical reactions are slight stinging in the mouth and increased salivation. Too much sour can lead to a sour disposition. Sour strengthens fluid and fire. It stimulates gastric fire, corrects digestive disorders. Sour is astringent, absorbent, and consolidating. The astringent taste falls under sour in Chinese medicine, conserving essence in the form of sweat, urine, semen, and diarrhea.

Excessive indulgence in the sour taste can result in upsetting blood composition, muscle weakness, inflammation, mouth ulcers, and any illness aggravated by an increase in fire.

Contraindications for sour are gastritis, internal bleeding, jaundice, and any disturbance of fire or water.

Sources of the sour flavor are sour fruits including hawthorne berry and schizandra, also oxalic-acid-containing vegetables such as spinach or chard.

ASTRINGENT

Astringency tends to be light, cold, and dry. Tannins create this flavor. Tannin causes proteins to precipitate out of fluid; this means that tissue shrinks when an astringent is applied. Astringency has an effect of focusing the energy. It is absorptive, normalizes skin pigmentation, and diminishes quantity of urine.

Astringency is used to treat diarrhea, premature ejaculation, breathing disorders, excess urination, and hemorrhage.

The excess astringent flavor can lead to heart pain, dry mouth, hoarse voice, constipation, impotence, lowered blood oxygenation, low spirits, debility, decay, joint pain, the tension of vessels and congestion of bodily fluids. Contraindications for astringency are general debility, dryness, and loss of appetite.

Typical astringent herbs are umeboshi plums, schizandra, and witch hazel.

SWEET

The sweet taste generates tissue. It is composed of sugars, carbohydrates, proteins, fats, and amino acids. This taste operates as a tonic if the channels are clear; if not, the bitter and pungent tastes must be used to regulate digestion and clear the channels.

The sweet taste strengthens memory, reduces the risk of abortion, and sooths burning sensations. It is very good in cases of debility.

Excessive sweet leads to obesity, ponderousness, loss of appetite, depressed immune system, increased colds, and flus. Contraindications are fluid retentive diseases, including colds and obesity.

Sources of the sweet flavor include grains, tonic herbs, dates, and licorice root.

CLOSING THE CIRCLE

The journey returns. In this book, I have attempted to convey my experience as a medical astrologer relative to cycles. As a tool for deepening the fundamental turn, I addressed the philosophical concerns of Daoism, alchemy, and a slight touch of early Greek and Indian humoral thought.

Not only philosophy, this work has seeds in practice. I use the cycles in medical astrology from the viewpoints of medical systems such as Ayurveda, chakra systems of India, Chinese medicine, alchemy, and new physics.

These cycles turn both ways and can be applied to the body with physical agents or to process with herbal medicine. Clockwise motions are diurnal rhythms and relate to the daily life, and the counterclockwise zodiacal motions are tied to larger issues of life purpose. This compass guides my clinical practice more fundamentally than any other astrological considerations.

APPENDIX I
GENERAL DIRECTIONALITY OF
PLANT PARTS

Arillus	Extension surrounding fruit	Down
Bulbus	Bulb	Down
Calyx	Leaf extensions at base of flower	Up
Caudex	Stem	Up
Caulis	Vine	Through
Concretio	Dry sap	Up and down
Cortex	Bark	Up and down
Lignum	Woody part	Up
Folium	Leaf	Up
Flos	Flower	Up
Fructus	Fruit	Down
Gemma	Sprout	Up
Herba	Whole plant	Up and down
Oleum	Oil	Down
Pedicellus	Stalk	Up and down
Pericarpium	Peel	Down
Pollen	Pollen	Out and down
Ramulus	Twig	Up and out
Radix	Root	Down
Rhizome	Root tendril	Down and out
Sanguis	Blood	Up and down
Sclerotium	Dense center of fungus	In
Secretio	Secretion	Up and down
Semen	Seed	Down
Spina	Thorn	Out
Succus	Sap, fresh	Up and down

APPENDIX II
DRACONIC AND CYCLE
EXAMPLE CHARTS

I selected the charts in this section using a convenience method. No attempt has been made to fit the chart to the method.

The Draconic method does not require high accuracy for birth data in the Rodden rating system. Reason: the 18.6-year draconic period of the Nodal axis provides the focal point for practice. Thus, time-sensitive points for errors will be the Moon, then Mercury, Venus and the Sun if they are close to a house cusp.

All charts are calculated using a tropical zodiac, which makes no difference since the techniques are not zodiac dependent. There is an exception, and that is the ascendant and the condition of its ruler for the cycle-based humoral analysis charts which follow the first three charts that demonstrate Draconic medicine.

Use the natalchart for constitutional assessment and risk assessment. I also use the draconic and cycle based techniques for consultation and decumbiture charts.

Figure 30

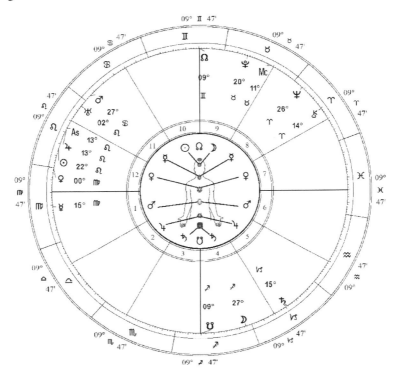

Draconic Method

Sri Aurobindo was a spiritual teacher who used writing as a feature of his spiritual discipline. His last days possessed a medical diagnosis of uremia (kidney failure). His passing was luminous and gentle, surrounded by the Mother and close disciples. Note Pluto in his third eye and the stellium of Jupiter, Sun, and Venus in his heart chakra. Saturn reduces energy in the second sexual chakra. Hands-on therapy, tuning forks for the planets and acupuncture are useful in the heart center, root chakra, and 3rd eye.

Figure 31

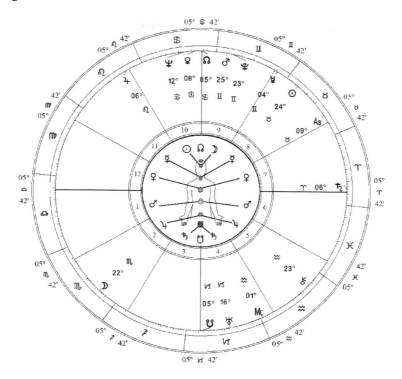

Draconic Method

Spiritual teacher Baba Muktananda has Neptune, Venus, Mars, and Pluto coalesced around the North Node of the Moon, which is the 6th chakra or the 3rd eye. His meditation techniques involved, in part, chanting and then moving into a meditative state where the 3rd eye opens into a blue field of light.

Figure 33

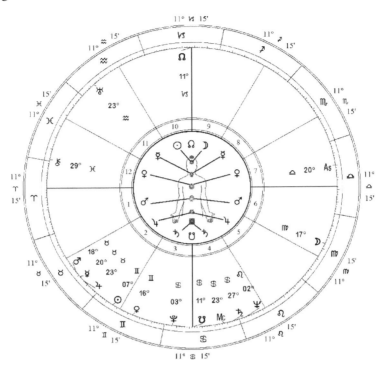

Draconic Method

John F. Kennedy was the 35th president of the United States of America. The planetary clusters around the South Node of the Moon are consistent with his low back problems. He received acupuncture and the use of Pluto, Saturn and Neptune tuning forks in the 3rd, 4th and 5th lumbar segments would have improved the results of the treatments that Janet Travel provided.

Figure 35

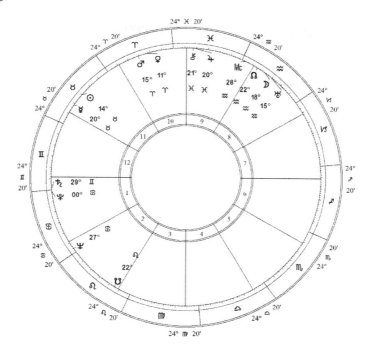

Day-Month-Year Cycle Analysis

Orson Welles is born in the springtime (warm-moist), mid-morning (warm-moist). Counting counterclockwise in zodiacal motion to discover the phase of the Moon, I begin at Taurus for the Sun and land on the Moon in Aquarius. Welles has a 4th quarter Moon which correlates with dry conditions. His ascendant is Gemini with cold-dry Saturn nearby. Mercury, the ruler of both the ascendant and Saturn, is in Taurus which is cold and dry. There would seem to be a preponderance of cold, dry melancholy as the ascendant's conditions easily overpower the background influences of the day-month-year cycles. There is, however, I must account for the warm-moist component for in dietary and herbal recommendations. A good distribution might be three parts warming and moistening strategies combined with two parts cooling and drying foods and medicinal.

Figure 36

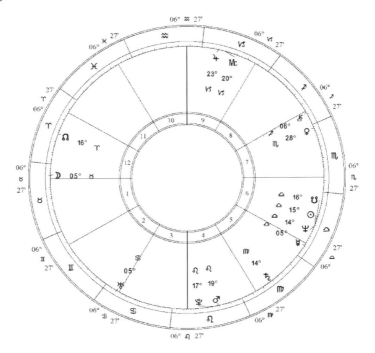

Day-Month-Year Cycle Analysis

Sigourney Weaver has Moon conjunct the ascendant, giving a damp signal. Venus rules the Asc and Moon; she is in Scorpio, giving a cold, wet influence. She is born in the fall just after sunset, both being in dry conditions. The Moon has just passed the opposition to the Sun, lending some warmth to the scenario. Dry and damp influences conflict with each other and harmonization is the treatment strategy – use both drying and moistening foods and herbs. There is a predominance of cold: Moon in Taurus, the ruler of Asc and Moon, Venus in Scorpio. Use warming agents while harmonizing moist and cold.

Figure 37

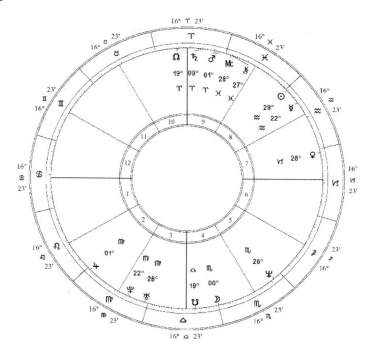

Day-Month-Year Cycle Analysis

Molly Ringwald is born mid-afternoon (hot and dry) in winter (cold and dry). She is born between a third and fourth quarter Moon (hot and dry). The Moon barely made it into Scorpio which is cold and wet, and the scant presence in Scorpio is fairly uncompelling to me. Nonetheless, her formula for food and herbs will be three parts moistening to one part drying with a balance of hot and cold agents.

APPENDIX III
AL BIRUNI ON MEDICINAL SUBSTANCES

This material is paraphrased from Ramesey Wright's 1934 translation of Al-Biruni's *Book of Instruction in the Elements of the Art of Astrology*. It is in the public domain and freely accessible [63, 64].

TREES & CROPS

Saturn comports with: oak-gall, citron, myrobalan, olive, willow, pine (turpentine), castor-oil plant. and all those which bear fruits with disagreeable taste or smell, or hard-shells such as walnuts and almonds, also sesame.

Jupiter comports with large trees and those that bear sweet fruit without hard skin such as peach, fig, apricot, pear and lote fruit.[56]

Venus comports with fruits and flowers: roses, sweet-smelling or tall, such plants as are light and whose seeds fly with the wind. Venus rules trees that are soft to the touch, sweet-smelling, smooth to the eye like cypress, teak, apple, and quince. Sweet and oily berries, fragrant and colored, herbs, spring flowers and has a share in cotton.

Mars resonates with trees that are bitter, pungent and thorny. Their fruit have rough skin, and they are pungent or very bitter such as bitter pomegranate, wild pear, bramble, mustard, leeks, onion, garlic, rue, radish, and eggplant.

---

[56] Lote fruit comes from the tree that marks the end of the seventh heaven, the boundary where no creation can pass, and beyond which is the Throne of Allah.

121

The Sun resonates with tall trees that have oily fruit such as date-palms, mulberries, dodder, sugarcane, and manna.

Mercury: pungent and evil-smelling trees, savory herbs and garden stuff, canes, and things growing in water.

The Moon: trees with short stems, vines and the sweet pomegranate. Also, grass, reeds, canes, flax, hemp, and trailing plants such as cucumber and melon.

METALS AND GEMS

Saturn: Litharge,[57] iron slag, hard stones, and lead.

Jupiter: Marcasite,[58] tutty,[59] sulphur, red arsenic, all white and yellow stones, stones found in ox-gall, tin, white lead, fine brass, diamond, all jewels worn by people.

Mars: Magnetic iron, cinnabar, rouge and mosaics, iron, and copper.

The Sun: Jacinths,[60] lapis lazuli, yellow sulphur, orpimem,[61] Pharaonic glass,[62] marble, realgar,[63] pitch, and gold.

Venus: Magnesia, antimony; silver, gold and jewels set in these; household vessels made of gold, silver, and brass, pearls, emeralds, and shells.

---

[57] Litharge is a lead monoxide
[58] Marcasite, is also called white iron pyrite, it is an iron sulfide.
[59] Tutty is a byproduct of brass production.
[60] Jacinth is a translucent red-orange variety of zircon often used as a gemstone.
[61] Orpinum is an orange-yellow stone composed of arsenic sulfide.
[62] The craft of glass making was introduced full-scale into Egypt by glass makers captured by Thutmose II (1479-1425 BC).
[63] Realgar is arsenic sulfide and is a reddish orange color.

Mercury: Depilatory,[64] arsenic, amber, all yellow and green stones, coins struck with name and number such as dinars, dirhams and coppers; old gold and quicksilver, turquoise, coral, and tree-coral.

The Moon: Nabatean glass, white stones, emerald, Moonstone; silver and things manufactured of silver, such as cups, bangles, rings and the like, pearls, crystal, and strung beads.

PLANT MATERIAL

Saturn: Pepper, belleric myrobalan, olives, hawthorn berries, bitter pomegranate, lentils, linseed, and hempseed.

Jupiter: Wild pomegranate, apple, wheat, barley, rice, durra, chick peas, sesame, and stones found in ox-gall.

Mars: Bitter almond and seed of turpentine-tree.

The Sun: Orange and maize.

Venus: Figs, grapes, dates, origanum, and fenugreek.

Mercury: Peas, beans, caraway, and coriander.

The Moon: Wheat, barley, large and small cucumbers, and melons.

FOOD & DRUGS

Saturn: Medicinals that are cold and dry in the fourth degree, especially those which are narcotic and poisonous. Sleep inducing agents and those that increase retentive power.

Jupiter: Those which are moderately hot and moist and are profitable and agreeable. Fruits. Those materials that increase

---

[64] Materials that can remove hair.

vitality and grow the nutritive faculties, and increase the air in the heart.[65]

Mars: Whatever is not poisonous but pungent and warm in the fourth degree.[66] Conventional medications are under Mars.

The Sun: Whatever is warm beyond the fourth degree and is salutary[67] and in general use.

Venus: Moderately cold and moist foods, useful and pleasant to the taste. Savory foods and herbs.

Mercury: Foods which are dryer than cold and are agreeable, but rarely useful, also grains.

The Moon: Foods which are equally cold and moist. Lunar foods are sometimes useful and sometimes detrimental. They are and are not in constant use as they can congest and cloy.

---

[65] Rhodeola is a great choice to improve 'air in the heart.' Greek Medicine sees the heart as being a location for the vital spirits, which it concentrates from *pneuma zoticon* which is sent from the lungs.

[66] Agents in the fourth degree are caustic and can burn the skin. These include many peppers and mustards.

[67] Salutatory is foods and activities that are generally health-promoting.

APPENDIX IV
HISTORY OF ENDOCRINE
SYSTEM THOUGHT

- Earliest discussion related to the endocrine system is attributed to English physician and gland specialist, Thomas Wharton (1614-1673), who distinguished between ductile and ductless glands [84]. Uranus was conjunct Neptune during this period.
- Dutch professor of anatomy and botany, Fredrik Ruysch (1638-1731) stated in 1690 that the thyroid secreted substances into the bloodstream [85]. Uranus was square Pluto at this juncture.
- French physician and animast/vitalist Theophile Bordeu (1722-1776) described body parts giving off emanations that influenced other areas of the body, in 1775 [86].
- German physiologist and zoologist Arnold Adolph Berthold (1803-1861), showed circulation of hormones in the blood in 1849, after castrating four chickens and then replanting the testes at different locations in two of the chickens, who then developed to maturity [87]. Uranus was conjunct Pluto by a wide 7-degree orb.
- The same year Berthold published his findings, Thomas Addison (1793-1860) identified Addison's disease [88]. Uranus was conjunct Pluto.
- Chinese medicine has reports of conditions called kidney yang and yin deficiencies as early as the late Han Dynasty (200 CE) [89, 90]. The patterns are transystemic and include the urinary tract, reproductive tract, central nervous system, hematopoietic system, and endocrine system. Kidney yang deficiency looks very much like hypothyroidism and kidney yin deficiency is close to hyperthyroidism. Uranus was sextile Pluto during this period.

APPENDIX V
GLOSSARY

Abstraction denotes the process of reducing information to a set of essential characteristics. It is the act of subsuming an observation into a broader level of generalization or logical order. For instance, classifying happiness as an emotional state reduces the amount of information conveyed about the emotional state.

Alchemy pertains to practices that are proto-chemistry in nature, but in this book, it refers to processes of transformation that are linked with synodic cycles.

Autonomy denotes the condition of being organizationally closed and self-referential.

Autopoiesis refers to a system capable of reproducing and maintaining itself. The term was introduced in 1972 by Chilean biologists Humberto Maturana and Francisco Varela to define the self-maintaining chemistry of living cells. Since then the concept has been also applied to the fields of cognition, systems theory, and sociology.

Blood denotes the physical blood in the body that moistens the muscles, tissues, skin, and hair and nourishes the cells and organs.

Channels denotes the pathways through which vitality flows to supply energy and nourishment to the body.

CHARTS

- Natal horoscope is the chart calculated for the birth of the native.
- Decumbiture refers to the chart calculated for the advent of a disease condition.

- The consultation chart is calculated for the moment of the consultation, it is a form of horary, and is also called interrogatory.
- The electional chart is used for timing the inception of a procedure, engaging in a program, or preparing a medicinal.
- Critical day charts are calculated for acute conditions upon the eightfold division of a lunar cycle. For chronic conditions, a chart is calculated for the moment of each 30 degrees of solar movement through the zodiac. They take forms of ingress charts.

Classical in this book denotes a premodern literature of the Classical period.

Cold denotes decreased functioning of an organ system and presents as any of the following: body aches, chills, poor circulation, fatigue, lack of appetite, loose stools or diarrhea, poor digestion, pain in the joints, slow movements and speech, aversion to cold, and craving for heat. Cold is present in all hypo conditions such as hypoadrenalism, hypoglycemia, and hypothyroidism.

Cosmobiology designates that branch of astrology working on scientific foundations and keyed to the natural sciences.

Damp denotes excessive fluids in the body with symptoms of abdominal bloating, loss of appetite, nausea, vomiting, lack of thirst, feeling of heaviness or being sluggish and stiff, aching or sore joints.

Damp heat denotes a condition of dampness and heat combined with symptoms of thick yellow secretions and phlegm such as jaundice, hepatitis, urinary problems, or eczema. It is one of the most common patterns for infection. The inflammation causes there to be redness and swelling, with condensation of fluids into thicker and darker accumulations of phlegm.

Dao denotes an ancient philosophy of 'the way' that provides a foundation for Chinese medical theory. Synonymous with Tao the word Dao is called a *pin yin* transliteration and it is the current academic and official standard of romanization. Tao is an earlier translational artifact from the Wade-Giles standard, which is not currently used in China, but still used in Taiwan for political reasons.

Deficiency denotes any weakness or insufficiency of qi, blood, yin, yang, or essence.

Draconic medicine pertains to the use of the nodal axis of the Moon as a tool for locating conditions and focusing treatment strategies. Draconic medicine assigns the length of the nodal axis to various segments of the anatomy for purposes of applying physical agents including sound, light, heat, cold, essential oils, acupressure, and acupuncture.

Dryness denotes a condition characterized by dry hair, lips, mouth, nose, skin, and throat, as well as extreme thirst and constipation.

Ecopsychosocial denotes a holistic worldview that includes the interior and exterior ecology and the psychological, spiritual and social experience.

Essence denotes substances that provides the basis of reproduction, growth, sexual power, conception, and pregnancy. It is the material foundation of qi and is stored in the kidneys. It is also referred to as *jing*.

Excess denotes an accumulation of food or vitality, and may include too much heat, cold, damp, yin or yang.

Existential (existentialism) denotes a philosophy of the 19th and 20th centuries that holds that because there are no universal values, man's essence is not predetermined, but based only on free choice; man is in a state of anxiety because of his realization of free will; and there is no objective truth. Major existentialists were Kierkegaard, Nietzsche, Sartre, Heidegger, Karl Jaspers, as well as the religious existentialists Martin Buber and Gabriel Marcel.

External denotes the location of illnesses, such as fevers and skin eruptions, on the surface of the body.

Fire can denote the result of the malfunction of the internal organs or can arise from extreme mood swings. Symptoms include fever, red or bloodshot eyes, swelling, sore throat, and flushed face. Fire may also present with dry mouth, bleeding or inflamed gums, or a desire for cold drinks.

Fractal denotes a rough or fragmented geometric shape that can be subdivided into parts, each of which is (at least approximately) a reduced-size copy of the whole.

Holism denotes the idea that all the properties of a given system (biological, chemical, social, economic, mental, linguistic, etc.) cannot be determined or explained by individual component parts. Instead, the system as a whole determines, in an important way, how the parts behave.

Humoral medicine denotes traditional medicines based upon environmental influences such as wind, heat, and damp.

Internal denotes the location of illnesses—such as those that affect the qi, blood, and organs—inside the body.

Microsystem denotes self-similar properties of biological systems, where the part is representative of the whole.

Paradigm denotes a thought pattern or epistemological context, a philosophical and theoretical framework or discipline used to compare and reveal through pattern identification; the term may also be used to describe evolving and transforming scientific ideologies.

Phlegm denotes a substance that may be visible and sticky, such as mucus, which can obstruct the channels, causing motor impairment and spasms. Phlegm is also used to describe muddled thinking and psychiatric disease characterized by extreme forms of cognitive incoherence.

Qi, pronounced [chee], is the vital energy or life-force, which flows through the meridians and is used to protect, transform, and warm the body. It is a term used throughout Chinese medicine to express a worldview based upon vitality. It might be useful to establish the functions of qi in a medical context in order to help define its use throughout this document. Qi warms, lifts, holds, and transforms. It commands blood. (This refers to the movement of the blood through the vessels). The lifting aspect of qi up-bears and is part of the energy that holds bodily structures and consciousness upright. Qi is a component of yang and warms. The qi function of warming is mild and physiologically normal, yet it also compels warmth in human interactions. The holding function of qi is that which maintains stability in both the function of the organs and the structures that hold the tissues in place. In opposition to the stable, holding function of qi is the transforming function of qi. The ability for the digestive system to transform foods into useable energy is an example. But, the transforming power of qi is also in the ability of individual, biological, and social systems to change. Supplementing qi and moving qi can assist each of these functions of qi.

Qigong [pronounced chee gung] denotes a set of exercises, including meditative and physical movements used to move qi, thereby maintaining or regaining physical, emotional, and spiritual health.

Recursion denotes the transformative recycling of a process. It is a process of feedback that involves a change in perspective.

Self-replicating system means a process by which a thing might make a copy of itself. For example, biological cells, given suitable environments, reproduce by division. Social systems also have tendencies towards self-replication.

Self-similarity, when applied to an object in mathematics, refers to an object exactly or approximately similar to a part of itself. This concept is applied in biological systems where a section will represent the whole.

Source pertains to origins. In Chinese medicine, there is a source within the kidneys that are embedded in the waters from which life arises. The beginning of a cycle is the source for synodic events.

Spirit is conscious, awake presence coursing through the blood vessels.

Stagnation denotes a blockage or buildup that prevents free flow. It is a precursor of illness and disease and is frequently accompanied by pain or tingling.

Systems are regularly interacting or interdependent group of objects that form an integrated whole. They are delimited by spatial and temporal boundaries. Open systems communicate and are influenced by the environment. Closed systems operate discretely.

Temporal denotes time and its influences, distinguished from space and relating to the sequence of time or to a particular time.

Tonification describes a therapeutic strategy used to nourish, support or strengthen a weakened condition of qi, blood or organ function.

Toxicity denotes any toxic load in the system that can be the result of exposure to toxins, byproducts of infection, or severe inflammatory diseases.

Transdisciplinarity refers to a unity of knowledge beyond disciplines, the existence of levels of reality, the logic of the included middle, and complexity. In the presence of several levels of reality, the space between disciplines and beyond disciplines is full of information.

Trans-systemic denotes a pattern of connections among systems.

Tropical-Sidereal Conundrum refers to the difference between two zodiacs. The tropical zodiac is based upon the seasonal features of the equinoxes and solstices. The sidereal zodiac uses the constellation of Aries as the starting point. Both zodiacs are abstractions of the sky. This difference poses a problem for astrology, which must be resolved as the gap between the two will eventually become 180^0 difference. Then, they will return in a grand time cycle of the Great Year at approximately 26,000 years.

Vibrational astrology (VA) is an approach to astrology that is systematic, evolving, and based upon rigorous evidence. It integrates ideas from several astrological systems (harmonic, symmetrical, humanistic, and Vedic) and modern physics, with innovations that are specific to VA.

Vitality denotes the continuous transformations that permeate the phenomenal world, unceasingly circulating, assembling, dispersing, converting, and making various combinations. The notion of vitality is bound within the paradox of life as a continuous unbroken field where discreet phenomenon are situated.

Yang denotes heat and the body's ability to generate and maintain warmth and circulation; it contributes to digestion, metabolism, and immune function. The Chinese character for yang represents the sunny side of a hill and the body's ability to generate and maintain warmth and circulation.

Yang deficiency denotes a cold condition due to lack of the heating quality of yang. Symptoms include lethargy, poor digestion, cold, lower back pain, and decreased sexual drive.

Yin denotes cool and the substance of the body, including blood and bodily fluids that nurture and moisten the organs and tissues. The Chinese character for yin represents the shady side of a hill.

Yin deficiency denotes a warm condition due to a lack of cooling, moistening functions. It results in symptoms of night sweats, fever, nervous exhaustion, dry eyes and throat, dizziness, blurred vision, insomnia, and a burning sensation in the palms of the hands, soles of the feet, and chest.

Zero point field denotes a unity field called the Wu Ji in Daoist thought.

REFERENCES

1. Jansky, R., *Astrology, Nutrition & Health.* 1977, Atglen, PA: Schiffer Publishing.
2. Popovic, M., *Reading the Human Body: Physiognomics and Astrology in the Dead Sea Scrolls and Hellenistic-Early Roman Period Judaism.* 2007: Brill.
3. Cox, J.C., *On a Ms. Calendar of the Fourteenth Century.* Reliquary: Archeological Journal and Review. 1888, London: Bemrose and Sons.
4. Curth, L., *The commercialisation of medicine in the popular press: English almanacs 1640-1700.* Seventeenth Century, 2002. **17**(1): p. 48-69.
5. Bocchi, G. and M. Ceruti, *The Narrative Universe* ed. A. Montouri. 2002, Cresskill, NJ: Hampton Press.
6. Gianluca Bocchi, E.C., Alfonso Montuori & Raffaella and Trigona, *History and Conditions for Creativity.* World Futures: The Journal of New Paradigm Research, 2014. **70**(5-6): p. 309-335.
7. Unschuld, P., *Medicine in China: a history of ideas.* 1985, Berkeley, CA: University of California Press.
8. Lehman, L., *Traditional Medical Astrology.* 2012: Schiffer Publishing, Ltd.
9. Campion, N., *The Traditional Revival in Modern Astrology: a Preliminary History.* Astrology Quarterly, Winter 2003. **74**(1): p. pp. 28-38.
10. Bateson, G., *Steps to an Ecology of Mind.* 1972, San Francisco: Chandler Publishing Company.
11. Unschuld, P.U., *Medicine in China: a history of ideas.* 1985, Berkeley,.
12. Unschuld, P., *Medicine in China, History Artifacts and Images.* 2000, Munich: Prestel Verlag.
13. Holden, J.H., *A History of Horoscopic Astrology.* 1996: American Federation of Astrologers, Inc.; 2nd edition.

14. Campion, N., *A History of Western Astrology Volume I: The Ancient and Classical Worlds* 2009: Bloomsbury Academic.

15. Reason, P., *A Participatory World.* Resurgence, 1998. **168**: p. 42-44.

16. Cesa, J. May 3, 1015]; Available from: http://commons. wikimedia.org/wiki/File:Celestial_equator_and_ecliptic.svg.

17. Bennett, N., *Foundations of Astrology.* 2014: BonAmi.

18. NASA. *Aero Space Dictionary.* [cited 2018 1/24]; Available from: https://www.hq.nasa.gov/office/hqlibrary/aerospace-dictionary/aerodictall/g.html.

19. Plofker, K., *Mathematics in India.* 2009: Princeton University Press.

20. Achar, N., *A Case for Revising the Date of the Vedanga Jyotisha.* Indian Journal of the History of Science, 2000. **35.3**: p. 173-183.

21. Hamilton, D.P.A., M. L. *The Astronomy Workshop.* 10/2000; Available from: http://adsabs.harvard.edu/abs/2000DPS....32.2505H.

22. Roman, E.M., et al., *The influence of the full moon on the number of admissions related to gastrointestinal bleeding.* Int J Nurs Pract, 2004. **10**(6): p. 292-6.

23. Chakraborty, U. and T. Ghosh, *A study on the physical fitness index, heart rate and blood pressure in different phases of lunar month on male human subjects.* International Journal of Biometeorology, 2013. **57**(5): p. 769-774.

24. Turanyi, C.Z., et al., *Association between lunar phase and sleep characteristics.* Sleep Med, 2014. **15**(11): p. 1411-6.

25. Wehr, T.A., *Bipolar mood cycles and lunar tidal cycles.* Mol Psychiatry, 2017.

26. Lee, K., et al., *Relationship between chronotype and temperament/character among university students.* Psychiatry Res, 2017. **251**: p. 63-68.

27. Unschuld, P., *Huang Di Nei Jing Su Wen: Nature, Knowledge, Imagery in an Ancient Chinese Medical Text.* 2003, Berkeley, CA: University of California Press.

28. Maturana, H. and F. Varela, *The Tree of Knowledge: A new look at the biological roots of human understanding*. 1986, Boston: New Science Library.
29. Humberto Maturana, F.V., *Autopoiesis and Cognition: The Realization of the Living*. Boston Studies in the Philosophy of Science. 1980: D. Reidel Publishing Company.
30. Pregadio, F., *jindan: Golden Elixir*, in *A Short Introduction to Chinese Alchemy*, H. Selin, Editor. 2007, Routledge: London.
31. Liu, H.-y., *Hui-ming Ching*. 1998 ed. 1793, Boston: Shambala.
32. Schmidt, R., *A Natural History of Time*, in *Phase Lecture Series*. 2004, The Golden Hind Press: Cumberland, Maryland.
33. Gebser, J., *The Ever-Present Origin*. 1949/1986, Athens, Ohio: Ohio University Press.
34. Ruiz, D.M. and J. Mills, *The Voice of Knowledge* 2013, San Rafael, California: Amber-Allen Publishing. pages cm.
35. Ruiz, D.M., Jr., *The five levels of attachment : toltec wisdom for the modern world*. 2013, San Antonio, VA: Hierophant Pub.
36. Crane, P., *Draconic Astrology*. 1987: Aquarian Press.
37. Lu, H., *A Complete Translation of the Nei Jing and Nan Jing: The Yellow Emperor's Classic*. 2004, Vancouver: International College of Traditional Chinese Medicine of Vancouver.
38. Jinsheng, P.U.U.a.H.T.w.Z., *Huang Di nei jing su wen: n Annotated Translation of Huang Di's Inner Classic – Basic Questions*. 2011, University of California Press. p. Chapters 1 through 52.
39. Bassingthwaighte, J.B., L.S. Liebovitch, and B.J. West, *Fractal Physiology*. 1994, New York: Oxford Press. i.
40. West, B.J., *Fractal Physiology and Chaos in Medicine (Studies of Nonlinear Phenomena in Life Science, Vol 1)*. 1991, Hackensack, NJ: World Scientific Pub Co Inc. pp21.
41. Wee, J.Z., *Discovery of the Zodiac Man in Cuneiform*. Journal of Cuneiform Studies, 2015. **67**.
42. Veith, I., *Huang ti nei ching su wên : the Yellow Emperor's classic of internal medicine : chapters 1-34 translated from the Chinese with an introductory study*. New ed. 1966, Berkeley: University of California Press. XXI,260 s.

43. Wang, B., *Yellow Emperor's Canon of Internal Medicine*, ed. A.Q.W. Nelson Liansheng Wu. 1997, Beijing: China Science and Technology Press.

44. Wu NL, W.A.T., *Yellow Emperor's Canon of Internal Medicine*. 1996, Shandong: China Science and Technology Press.

45. Wu and Wu, *Yellow Emperor's Canon of Internal Medicine*. 1996, Beijing: China Science and Technology Press.

46. Davidson, W.M., *Davidson's Medical Astrology: A Series of Eight Lectures on Medical Astrology and Health*. 1959, Monroe, New York: Astrological Bureau

47. Witte, A., *Regelwerk für Planetenbilder*. 1928, Hamburg, Germany: Ludwig Rudolph Verlag.

48. Witte, A., *Der Mensch*. 1975, Hamburg, Germany: Ludwig Rudolph Verlag.

49. Ebertin, R., *Combination of Stellar Influences*. 1972, Aalen, Germany,: Ebertin-Verlag.

50. Zhang, Y., *ECIWO biology and medicine: A new theory of conquering cancer and a completely new acupuncture therapy*. 1987: Neimenggu People's Press.

51. Schjelderup, V., *ECIWO biology and medicine: A new theory of conquering cancer and a completely new acupuncture therapy*. Acupuncture in Medicine, 1992.

52. Woodroffe, J., *The Serpent Power: Being the Sat-Cakra-Nirupana and Paduka-Pancaka*. 1973: Ganesh & Co.

53. Leadbeater, C.W., *The Chakras: A MONOGRAPH* 2009: Anand Gholap Theosophical Institute.

54. Lazarev, N.V. in *7th All- union Congr. Physiol., Biochem., Pharmacol*. 1947. Medgiz, Moscow.

55. Langevin, H.M., et al., *Connecting (T)issues: How Research in Fascia Biology Can Impact Integrative Oncology*. Cancer Research, 2016. **76**(21): p. 6159-6162.

56. Aristotle; Stocks, J.L.J.L., 1882-1937; Wallis, Harry Bernard, *De caelo* 1922, Oxford: The Clarendon Press.

57. Levin, F., *The Manual of Harmonics of Nichomachus the Pythagorean*. 1994: Phanes Press.

58. Zeyl, D.a.S., Barbara, *The Stanford Encyclopedia of Philosophy* Plato's Timaeus, ed. E.N. Zalta. 2017, : Metaphysics Research Lab, Stanford University.

59. Custo, H., *The Cosmic Octave: Origin of Harmony*. 2015: LifeRhythm

60. Colbert, A.P., et al., *Magnets applied to acupuncture points as therapy – a literature review*. Acupuncture in Medicine, 2008. **26**(3): p. 160-170.

61. Erlewine, M., *Local Space Relocation Astrology*. 2006, Big Rapids, Michigan: StarTypes.com.

62. Lilly, W., *Christian Astrology*. 3rd ed. 1985, Exeter: Regulus.

63. Biruni, A., *Book of Instruction in the Elements of the Art of Astrology*. 2006: Astrology Classics

64. Biruni, A., *The Book of Instruction in the. Elements of Astrology*. 1934, London: Luzac & Co.

65. Light, P.D., *Southern Folk Medicine: Healing Traditions from the Appalachian Fields and Forests*. 2018: North Atlantic Books.

66. Greenbaum, D.G., *Temperament - Astrology's Forgotten Key*. 2005: The Wessex Astrologer Ltd.

67. Culpeper, N., *Astrological Judgment of Disease from the Decumbiture of the Sick*. 1655: Ascella.

68. Culpeper, N., *English Physician*, in *Culpeper's Complete Herbal: A Book of Natural Remedies for Ancient Ills*. 1880, Foulshom: London.

69. Thulesius, O., *Nicholas Culpeper English Physician and Astrologer*. 1992: St. Martin's Press.

70. Tobyn, G., *Culpeper's Medicine: A Practice of Western Holistic Medicine*. 1997, Rockport, MA: Element Books.

71. Lilly, W., *1-3: Christian Astrology (Three Volumes in One)*. 2011: Cosimo Classics

72. Hill, J., *Medical Astrology: A Guide to Planetary Pathology* 2004: Stellium Press.

73. Hoffman, O., *Classical Medical Astrology - Healing with the Elements*. 2009: The Wessex Astrologer Ltd

74. Tulku, T., *Love of knowledge*. 1984, Berkeley, CA: Dharma Press.

75. Sydenham, T., *The Works of Thomas Sydenham, M.D.* . Reprint of the 1848 and 1850 London Sydenham Society volumes 1 and 2 ed. 1979, Birmingham Alabama: Classics of Medicine Library

76. Foucault, M., *The Birth of the Clinic: an Archaeology of Medical Perception*. World of man. 1973, New York,: Pantheon Books. 215.

77. Rudhyar, D., *The Lunation Cycle: A Key to the Understanding of Personality*. 1967, Santa Fe, NM: Aurora Press.

78. Kranich, E.M., *Planetary Influences Upon Plants: A Cosmological Botany*. 1984, Wyoming, Rhode Island: Bio – Dynamic Literature.

79. Steiner, R., *Die Polaritat von Dauer und Entwicklung im Menschenleben GA 184*. 1968: Dornach.

80. Goethe, J.W.v., *The Metamorphisis of Plants*. 2009, Cambridge, Massachusetts: The MIT Press.

81. Shiva, V., *Monocultures of the Mind: Biodiversity, Biotechnology and Agriculture*. 1993, New Delhi: Zed Press.

82. Henry Cornelius Agrippa, K., *Three Books of Occult Philosophy, or of Magick*.

83. Lilly, W. 3rd ed. 1985, Exeter: Regulus.

84. Sawin, C.T., *Historical Note: Thomas Wharton (1614-1673) and the Glands of the Body*. The Endocrinologist, 2000. **10**(5): p. 283&hyhen;288.

85. Boer, L., A.B. Radziun, and R.J. Oostra, *Frederik Ruysch (1638–1731): Historical perspective and contemporary analysis of his teratological legacy*. American Journal of Medical Genetics. Part a, 2017. **173**(1): p. 16-41.

86. Dominique, B., *THE MEDICAL PHILOSOPHY OF THEOPHILE DE BORDEU (1722-1776)*. 2004, Paris: Honore Champion.

87. Loriaux, D.L., *Arnold Adolph Berthold (1803–1861)*, in *A Biographical History of Endocrinology*. 2016, John Wiley & Sons, Ltd. p. 91-96.

88. Pearce, J.M.S., *Thomas Addison (1793-1860)*. Journal of the Royal Society of Medicine, 2004. **97**(6): p. 297-300.

89. Yunbai [柯勻伯] , K. and K. Qin [柯琴] , *Collection of Cold Damage for Revival [Shāng Hán Lái Sū Jí,* 傷寒來蘇集*]*. 1674 Qīng (清) dynasty.

90. Zhang, Z., et al., *Shang Han Lun: On Cold Damage, Translation and Commentaries*. 1999, Boulder, CO: Paradigm Publications.

Made in the USA
San Bernardino, CA
17 July 2019